Quality, Evidence and Effectiveness in Health Promotion

Health promotion specialists have long grappled with how to measure the quality and effectiveness of their research and practice. This is the first book to combine these two concepts in one volume.

The book addresses:

- research effectiveness through the examination of different evaluative methodologies
- practice-based quality assurance programmes
- examples of health promotion interventions which work.

Quality, Evidence and Effectiveness in Health Promotion attempts to demonstrate that health promotion is a crucial area for investment by policymakers. The book will be invaluable to practitioners, academics and students working in health promotion and public health.

John Kenneth Davies is Senior Lecturer in Health Promotion at the University of Brighton; **Gordon Macdonald** is Professor of Health Promotion Policy and Development at the University of Glamorgan.

Quality, Evidence and Effectiveness in Health Promotion

Striving for certainties

Edited by John Kenneth Davies
and Gordon Macdonald

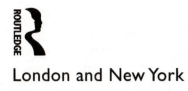

London and New York

First published 1998
by Routledge
11 New Fetter Lane, London EC4P 4EE

Simultaneously published in the USA and Canada
by Routledge
29 West 35th Street, New York, NY 10001

Typeset in Garamond by
Ponting–Green Publishing Services, Chesham, Buckinghamshire
Printed and bound in Great Britain by
Creative Print & Design (Wales), Ebbw Vale

British Library Cataloguing in Publication Data
A catalogue record for this book is available
from the British Library.

Library of Congress Cataloging in Publication Data
Quality, Evidence and Effectiveness in Health Promotion / edited by
John Kenneth Davies and Gordon Macdonald.
    p.   cm.
  Includes bibliographical references and index.
  1. Health promotion.
  I. Davies, John K. (John Kenneth).
  II. Macdonald, Gordon
  RA427.8.Q35   1998
  613–dc21   98–22995
  CIP

ISBN 0–415–17966–1 (hbk)
ISBN 0–415–17967–X (pbk)

Contents

Figures

Tables

Contributors

Frances Baum is Associate Professor and Head of the Department of Public Health, Flinders University of South Australia and Director of the South Australia Community Health Research Unit in Adelaide, Australia.

Noreen M. Clark is Dean and Marshall H. Becker Professor of Public Health in the School of Public Health at the University of Michigan, USA.

John Kenneth Davies is Senior Lecturer in Health Promotion and Course Director of the Masters in Health Promotion (Europe) in the School of Applied Social Science, Faculty of Health at the University of Brighton, England.

Alain Deccache is Professor and Director of the Health Education Unit (RESO) in the School of Public Health at the Catholic University of Louvain, Brussels, Belgium.

Bo J.A. Haglund is Professor in Public Health Sciences and Director of the WHO Collaborating Centre on Supportive Environments for Health, Karolinska Institute, Stockholm, Sweden.

Bjarne Jansson is Associate Professor in Community Medicine and Course Director of the Masters in Public Health Education at the Karolinska Institute, Stockholm, Sweden.

Jolanda F.E.M. Keijsers is a Quality Manager at the Dutch Institute for Health Promotion and Disease Prevention, Woerden, The Netherlands.

Cecily Kelleher is Professor of Health Promotion and Director of the Centre for Health Promotion Studies at University College, Galway, Ireland.

Ilona Kickbusch is Director of the Division for Health Promotion, Education and Communication, World Health Organisation Headquarters, Geneva, Switzerland.

Jean Laperche is a general medical practitioner and Director of the FMMCSF

(Fédération des Maisons Médicales et Collectifs de Santé Francophones) Health Promotion Project, Brussels, Belgium.

Gordon Macdonald is Professor of Health Promotion Policy and Development at the Welsh Institute for Health and Social Care at the University of Glamorgan, Wales.

Kenneth R. McLeroy is Professor and Chair of the Department of Health Promotion Sciences at the University of Oklahoma College of Public Health, USA.

Bosse Pettersson is Director of the Swedish National Institute for Public Health and Senior Lecturer, Masters of Public Health programme, Department of Public Health Sciences, Karolinska Institute, Stockholm, Sweden.

Liz Rogers is a researcher and trainer in the Health Promotion Division of the Wessex Institute for Health Research and Development, University of Southampton, England.

Irving Rootman is Director of the Centre for Health Promotion at the University of Toronto, Canada.

Annette Rushmere is a researcher in the Health Promotion Division of the Wessex Institute for Health Research and Development, University of Southampton, England.

J.A.M. Saan is a senior consultant on quality, policy and strategy at the Dutch Centre for Health Promotion and Disease Prevention, Woerden, The Netherlands.

Viv Speller is Senior Lecturer and Director of the Health Promotion Division of the Wessex Institute for Health Research and Development, University of Southampton, England.

Jane Springett is Professor of Health Promotion and Public Health, Institute of Health, Liverpool John Moores University, England.

Per Tillgren is Director of the Health Education course at the Karolinska Institute, Stockholm, Sweden.

Erio Ziglio is Responsible Officer for the Health Promotion and Investment Programme at the World Health Organisation Regional Office for Europe in Copenhagen, Denmark.

Foreword

The pressure to prove that 'health promotion works' is particularly strong at this point in time when health care reforms call for never ending streams of evidence, efficiency and effectiveness measures, frequently defined by a marriage of convenience between economic rationalism and clinical outcome.

Health promotion measures its impact and outcome with quite a different tool box. This book, the first with such a comprehensive content, surveys the evaluation processes and methods and discusses the challenges that quality assurance in health promotion presents. Some practical examples are offered which give both academics and practitioners an opportunity to review aspects of quality and effectiveness on a global scale.

Health promotion constitutes a change in perspective and paradigm, since it challenges both conceptual frameworks and methods of intervention. It is challenged in turn to prove that 'it works': in many cases, with more than established clinical and management procedures. This book accepts the challenge and provides professionals in the field of health promotion with supportive evidence.

The World Health Organization also recognises the uncertainty that such change brings. It works with partners around the world – in particular its strong network of collaborating centres – to strengthen the knowledge base for health promotion interventions so as to ensure their quality and effectiveness. The challenges raised by health promotion enable us to move the field of public health forward: the uncertainties of today carry the seeds of the solutions of tomorrow.

This book will prove as useful for those practising health promotion as for those who are involved in health promotion research and teaching. In particular though, I would hope that policy-makers, decision-makers and critics of health promotion find time to study it. They will discover much food for thought – and hopefully a reason to invest in health promotion on a larger scale, moving it from the margins to the centre of the playing field.

Ilona Kickbusch PhD
Director, Division of Health Promotion
Education and Communication
World Health Organization Headquarters

Preface

The original idea and impetus for this book came from the editors' work as members of the Scientific Planning Committee for the Third European Conference on Effectiveness: Quality Assessment in Health Promotion and Health Education, held in Turin in September 1996. This conference highlighted the more general concern that health promotion was increasingly needing to justify itself and its use of scarce resources. In particular it needed to apply appropriate processes for quality assurance and more rigorous measures of effectiveness. Many of the contributors to this volume participated in the conference and were involved in identifying similar concerns, 'grappling with the uncertainties' involved and discussing possible solutions. This reflected the importance of this event and its catalytic effect internationally, in terms of the future direction of quality improvement and evidence-based practice in health promotion.

The book therefore provides researchers, practitioners and policy-makers with a unique, state of the art publication on quality assurance and evaluation in health promotion globally. Although it critiques conventional approaches to evaluation, it doesn't pretend to have simple alternatives. Instead it offers a valuable aid to critical analysis, drawing on the ideas of some of the foremost international thinkers in this key area of health and social development.

This book would not have come to fruition without the assistance, both intellectual and practical, of many people. We wish to acknowledge the advice and support of all members of the Scientific Committee of the 1996 Turin Conference, particularly Professor Lamberto Briziarelli, University of Perugia, and Dr Mario Carzana, Piemonte Regione, in the initial preparation of the book. Thanks are also due to other colleagues from Piemonte Regione and from the Italian Committee for Health Education. In addition, many thanks to Heather Gibson and Fiona Bailey at Routledge for their help and support during the preparation of this volume. Finally, and not least, we wish to acknowledge the administrative support of the University of Brighton, particularly the assistance of Eleanor James, Jean Ross and Janice Lyons, in preparation of the final manuscript.

John Kenneth Davies and Gordon Macdonald
Brighton and Cardiff
June 1998

Introduction

Gordon Macdonald and John Kenneth Davies

The key concerns that arose during the European Conference on Effectiveness in Turin in 1996 focused around three key issues.

First, if health promotion is to remain at the forefront of local, national and international health policy development and investment, it needs to establish, as a matter of some urgency, a framework for evidence-based practice. This framework would not only include reference to established and conventional research methods, which help prove the effectiveness of interventions, but also incorporate more developmental evaluative methods that aid the understanding of the progress and process of an intervention's life as well as its outcome.

Second, there is a growing realisation that traditional logical positivist approaches to health promotion research and evaluation no longer provide the right questions (or indeed answers) for many health promotion interventions. These approaches tend to be rooted firmly in the biomedical model and the origins of *disease*, which, although the mainstay of many early health promotion research programmes, are now having to give way to more pluralist, postmodernist approaches, based on the origins of *health*. Only by encouraging this development can health promoters discover the answers to the 'how' and 'why' of programmes as well as the 'what' and 'when'. In practice this will involve using the best of both research paradigms and methods in a form of triangulation, such that it will provide epistemological validity and reliability. The chapters in this volume support this trend towards non-positivist approaches to research. It is heartening to note that others are now responding to this call for broadening the base to research, including in England, a Health Education Authority sponsored working group on evidence in health promotion.

Third, and more recently, specialists in health promotion and public health are attempting to gain an understanding of the whole process of quality assurance (QA) and how it applies to their work in order to improve practice. Various options that include Continuous Quality Improvement, Total Quality Management, External Standards Inspection and others, have all contributed to a feeling that there is a need to monitor and audit health promotion work to help develop best practice. This again, is probably achieved through some kind of process quality audit combined with standards setting, using indicators and criteria, which together, produce a comprehensive QA programme.

These concerns are inevitably linked, the second and third issues providing the mechanism and detail to help inform the larger framework for evidence-based practice. It is also true that the kinds of debate going on between the two research paradigms are being mirrored in emerging discussions on quality assurance. QA programmes, like sound and beneficial research, must provide answers to process (and input) variables in programme development and implementation, and not concentrate on the impact and outcome of interventions. This embryonic consensus on research methodology and QA approaches is evident in this book.

The book is nominally divided into three parts which reflect the themes in the title. The first part looks specifically at examples of methods for assessing evidence and effectiveness with contributions from the United States, Ireland and Australia. The Clark and McLeroy paper (chapter 2), which is rooted in health promotion developments in the United States, provides a comprehensive account of the models and concepts that should and do underpin the evolving knowledge base of health promotion. Whilst many of these models are drawn from psychological theories on behaviour change, there is an acknowledgement that other theories are essential for more broadly-based health promotion practice. Theories which form socio-ecological, environmental and empowerment approaches to the promotion of health are critical starting points for broader based evidence work. They help to explain the settings approach to health promotion, which is also considered in this chapter, and the trend towards consumer power. Kelleher elaborates on the settings approach in chapter 3. She describes and discusses public health programmes in four key settings in Ireland. The school, workplace, primary health care and the community all lend themselves to health promotion interventions, but as Kelleher stresses, the evidence to effect change beyond the individual, remains somewhat illusory. However the chapter concludes that uncertainty should not be an excuse for inaction. We need to test interventions on the best available evidence, the author argues, and not wait for certainties.

The third chapter in the first part of the book, highlights an approach to effectiveness in one setting, the community. Although based on experiences in Australia, Baum draws on literature from around the globe to support her view that community approaches, based on principles of participation and empowerment, offer real alternatives to traditional individual lifestyle approaches, so evident in the 1970s and 1980s. But because concepts of empowerment and participation can be contentious and ill-defined, evaluation of community based programmes can cause problems. Baum helps by provides the reader with a useful evaluation checklist based on participatory action research.

The second part of the book examines the issue of quality assessment and provides concrete examples of how quality issues can be made more applicable through the use of appropriate instruments and guidelines. Chapter 5 from Sweden builds on work first developed at the Sundsval Conference in 1991. Haglund, Jansson, Pettersson and Tillgren provide an easily understood 20-item instrument for assessing the quality of an intervention. This work is complemented by Keijsers and Saan who, in their chapter, report on two alternative instruments (Analys and Preffi) used in the Netherlands. These instruments assess first the quality of the research methodology applied to health promotion interventions (Analys) and second the quality of practice by health promotion specialists (Preffi). Both these chapters provide useful and practical tools for researchers and practitioners to assess the quality of their work with a little more certainty.

The chapter by Speller, Rogers and Rushmere (7) describes two pieces of work which again contribute to health promotion practice. The QA manuals on standards for practice and healthy alliances are both in use in the UK. Three examples of schemes or initiatives that have applied quality standards are described. The authors conclude that their work could form the basis for further developments in QA in health promotion which could then be subject to vigorous effectiveness testing.

The third and final part of the book includes three chapters which attempt to synergise aspects of effectiveness with aspects of quality assurance. Chapter 8 (Deccache and Laperche) revisits the theoretical bases to evaluative research and quality assurance. It then provides an interesting case study of the development of a quality assessment system for primary health care in Belgium. The authors point out that the relevance of health promotion activity should take precedence over scientific complexity or political necessity. The primary health care project in Belgium attempted to make health promotion relevant by involving the users in the aims and outcomes of the project,

In chapter 9, Springett examines in some detail the issues that faced Liverpool in the UK when it attempted to implement the key features of the Health For All programme at city level. In particular she describes and analyses the ways alternative forms of evaluation can contribute to the processes of public policy development. In turn she argues that health policy can help develop evaluative techniques for quality assurance.

Chapter 10 by Rootman and Ziglio provides readers with an international perspective of current work around quality assurance and effectiveness. The authors describe the deliberations of a WHO working group as it grappled with new ideas and their application to practice. Much of the work described in this chapter is to be published in a forthcoming WHO monograph and this should help promote a dialogue between WHO and others working in the same area.

The final chapter revisits and extends our opening chapter 1. If effectiveness and evidence-based practice are to lead the new health promotion paradigm as it embraces alternative evaluative research methodologies, then it needs clear direction. The chapter sets out a seven step plan leading towards a more post-modern approach to effectiveness and quality assessment that seeks to place health promotion at the heart of investment in public health and health care in the twenty-first century. It is an attempt to get ideas on evaluation and quality moving towards a new paradigm for a new century.

Chapter 1

Reflection and vision

Proving and improving the promotion of health

Gordon Macdonald and John Kenneth Davies

INTRODUCTION

Health promotion has matured rapidly in the last quarter of the twentieth century. From rather humble and embryonic beginnings in the late 1960s, characterised by a search for disciplinary roots and an acceptable theoretical base, it has blossomed and flourished into an international discipline and practice and found itself at the forefront of the new public health movement. Despite this meteoric rise and the accompanying trans-national attention it has received, it is still a relatively new discipline, and as such struggles to establish itself along side the more traditional and the more accepted disciplines like education, medicine and psychology (Macdonald and Bunton 1993). Major influential initiatives such as Health For All, the Alma Ata Declaration, and the Healthy Cities programme have helped raise the profile of health promotion, but substantial doubts remain about its effectiveness and its value in tackling the major issues affecting population health (Williams and Popay 1994, Peberdy 1997).

This chapter will provide a conceptual framework for the book by tracing, briefly, the development of health promotion since the 1960s. By examining first its theoretical roots and the struggle for conceptual supremacy, the chapter will continue by looking back to *reflect* on effectiveness and effectiveness studies as a way of *proving* the value of health promotion in reducing premature death and disability and promoting health. But it will also look forward for a *vision* of the future based on a quality assurance approach to *improve* practice. It will therefore be both reflective and visionary in its attempt to *strive towards certainties* in the field of health promotion theory and practice.

ROOTS OF HEALTH PROMOTION

Agreement is needed now on the knowledge base for health promotion in order to provide appropriate evidence, demonstrate effectiveness and improve quality. This knowledge base will underpin health promotion theory and practice, including consideration of key issues such as ideology, value systems, methodologies, measurement instruments and indicators.

Only when we are clear on these fundamental issues can we begin to attempt to *prove* effectiveness and recommend a quality assurance process to *improve* health promotion. We will return to these two areas later, but first we want to trace the knowledge base and the conceptual roots of health promotion.

One of the earlier approaches to the promotion of health was based on education and psychology. The educational approach, although used pragmatically from the early part of the present century, is essentially a tool of preventive medicine. Dominated by a biomedical risk factor paradigm, it is based on a social regulationist approach (Caplan 1993), which assumes that change can be brought about within society's existing regulatory structures primarily by modifying individual behaviours. From the 1950s onwards, the theory and practice of health education developed in the United States, through the establishment of individual and social psychological models of health-related knowledge, attitude and behaviour change. Underlying this approach are positivist-empiricist principles from natural science, which assume that people are rational and logical in the way they behave. Evidence of the effectiveness of such interventions rely firmly on short-term outcomes using empirical data linked to knowledge, attitude and/or behaviour change.

Health promotion grew rapidly during the 1980s and reflected a paradigm shift from an individual focus on medical problems to a broader structuralist approach which included environmental, economic, socio-cultural and legislative measures to promote health (WHO 1984). It has developed from dissatisfaction with the professionally dominant, individual change paradigm and a realisation of its limitations. It conceives health as occurring within a complex system of variables, incorporating individual biomedical and psychological factors within a socio-ecological and environmental context. Bennett and Murphy (1997) argue that, although psychological theories have proved useful in motivating and maintaining behaviour change in the community, there is a need for health promotion programmes to change focus from individual behaviour change alone to incorporate more structural alterations.

Health promotion has been defined as: 'the *process* of enabling people to increase *control* over, and to improve, their health' (WHO 1986).

The key concepts in this definition are 'process' and 'control'; and therefore effectiveness and quality assurance in health promotion must focus on enabling and empowerment (Dreber 1996). If the activity under consideration is not enabling and empowering then it is not health promotion (Ziglio 1996). These concepts are reflected in the action areas of the Ottawa Charter for Health Promotion (WHO 1986), which fundamentally advocates a basic change in the way society is organised and resources distributed. Many of these structural changes relate to different concepts of community, which is traditionally seen as a population or a large group of disparate individuals to be targeted, through the mass media for example. Health promotion perceives community as a setting or a form of social system or network that has the potential to act as a resource to promote health 'ecologically' from the bottom up. Community members identify and express their own needs and participative, community development strategies are negotiated with health promoters. The values which underpin this approach are based on 'Health for All' principles of participation, empowerment, sustainability and a desire for equity in health (WHO 1978). The vehicles operationalising this approach to health promotion are based on settings, where people live and work, such as Healthy Cities, Health Promoting Schools, Health Promoting Hospitals and Healthy Workplaces. Its programmes are multi-level and include diverse yet complementary activities such as developing individual resources and social skills, strengthening community action and creating healthy public policy. Its conceptual robustness and value-added dimension relies on these diverse activities operating synergistically to promote health. It is the understanding of such processes that facilitates synergy and their interrelationship with health gain, that is central to health promotion.

However, because of the 'newness' of the subject the history of the development of health promotion has been one of promoting the subject through a form of missionary zeal and evangelism. This approach, epitomised by a subscription to symposia statements with rhetoric that reflects the desire to be taken seriously, coupled with programme developments that expand horizontally rather than vertically, has been necessary because the crucial issue has been profile and agenda setting. Statements from Ottawa (WHO 1986), Adelaide (WHO 1988), Sundsvall (WHO 1991) and Jakarta (WHO 1997) have all advocated the core or central role health promotion can and must play in the drive to improve health nationally and internationally.

Additionally programmes based on settings as cited above, such as the Healthy Cities (HCs) movement and the Health Promoting Schools (HPS) initiative, have striven for horizontal expansion (recruitment to the network). It is the case for example, that the HCs project now has 34 project cities in Europe alone and some 250 worldwide (Springett 1998) and the HPS has some 500 core schools in 40 European countries (HEA 1997). This horizontal expansion is at the real expense of vertical development (deepening the programme) in a more limited number of cities and schools. This would have allowed an understanding of the process of programme and intervention development, which in turn would have enhanced the capacity to monitor and evaluate effectiveness.

Second, the statements which come out of Ottawa or Jakarta are important but they provide ammunition for the health promotion sceptics who might argue that the subject tries too hard to be all things to all people. Statements which argue for the abolition of war and poverty because they are the biggest contributors to ill health are naive in the extreme and only mimic other grandiose conference statements concerned with population growth, social conditions or conflict resolution. Health promotion declarations and statements need to confine themselves to locating health within a larger social whole, but they need to reflect a rigorous theoretical research base that is designed to improve practice and make it more effective.

EFFECTIVENESS AND EVALUATION

This need to raise the profile of health promotion through programme expansion at the national and international levels has in many ways clouded clear approaches to evaluation and evidence of effectiveness. This is rather ironic given the 'lead' that health education and later, health promotion, gave in the quest for appropriate and suitable evaluation tools (Macdonald 1996). Earlier debates in health promotion were often surrounded by the call to consider the right methodology to evaluate the intervention (Gatherer *et al.* 1979, Green and Lewis 1986, Means and Smith 1988). It might be that in some ways, health promotion has suffered, from its self-inflicted demand to consider evaluative methods, by being too ambitious. Many of the evaluation techniques were based on an unrealistic idea of what health promotion could or even should achieve and were largely concerned with outcome data. This traditional biomedical approach to evaluation has received a great deal of criticism in recent years, and a consensus is undoubtedly emerging that an over concentration on outcome measures and indeed on quantitative data, is an outmoded and inappropriate way to measure the effectiveness of health promotion programmes and interventions (Nutbeam 1996, Allensworth 1994). This consensus is reflected in this volume. Lipsey *et al.* (1985) were among the first to identify the inherent problems of trying to evaluate the effectiveness of health promotion programmes through the adoption of experimental designs for research. They argued that because health promotion took place within a natural and complex setting (the community or society) it was impossible, even if desirable, to control for all the variables that might affect health. Further, they proposed that traditionally trained evaluators (biomedical researchers) might not be sufficiently skilled to carry out more pragmatic approaches to design given the increasingly naturalistic 'field' conditions.

This concern has been mirrored in more recent criticisms of the biomedical outcomes model of evaluation (Baum 1988, Raeburn 1992, Hepworth 1997). Essentially what the critics are arguing is that health promotion programmes and interventions need to be assessed in relation to the social and structural influences that determine health. They therefore need to adopt an approach to evaluation that implicitly acknowledges the need for outcome data but explicitly concentrates on process or illuminative data that helps us understand the nature of that relationship. This approach to evaluative research that recognises 'people variables' and natural settings within the community has been applied to some interesting and testing case studies (Allison and Rootman 1996, Costongs and Springett 1997).

Within the current contract culture however, priority is given to practices that emphasise measurable outcomes (Ovretveit 1996). Centres being established to study evidence-based health (medical) care rely on the biomedical, logical-positivist paradigm, epitomised in the randomised control trial. Such centres require evidence utilising quantitative and empirical criteria (Sheldon *et al.* 1993). Health promotion finds this problematic and uncomfortable (Burrows 1996). It is often impossible to demonstrate causal links due to the complex interplay of variables. There are also inevitable time lags related to health status outcomes, which are often inter-generational.

Health promotion evaluative methodologies designed to measure effectiveness, unlike methods in other evidence-based health care interventions, have to consider how to gain an understanding of the processes involved in the planning and implementation of a programme. They also need to assess the impact the social and physical environment has on the programme. Process evaluation which may employ qualitative methods can offer critical and illuminating evidence of what happens during a programme's life (Macdonald *et al.* 1996). If we want to find out why a programme has achieved its goals and objectives or not, rather than whether it has, process or illuminative research should provide the answers.

Further, evaluation of large-scale health promotion programmes, such as the Healthy Cities movement (Davies and Kelly 1993) and Heartbeat Wales (Nutbeam *et al.* 1993), has proved difficult. This has been mainly due to the difficulty of isolating environmental and multimodal intervention effects and assessing their impact on health status outcomes. It has been suggested that even the processes of dissemination of such programmes through communities should be legitimate outcome targets for health promotion (Nutbeam *et al.* 1993). These may be termed 'intermediate outputs' (Whelan *et al.* 1993) or intermediate indicators, but are also useful process indicators. In this sense it is important for researchers in health promotion to acknowledge that their own training and disciplinary background along with their own value system will, to some extent, determine their approach to research methodology. With the new millennium there is a discernible movement towards the process and illuminative evaluative method. This will undoubtedly mean shifting the goal posts and refocusing on new measures of achievement. We would like to illustrate this by providing three examples of approaches to effectiveness that demonstrate an ability to respond to the need for an innovative way to consider health promotion and evaluation.

Intermediate indicators of success

It might be the case that conventional use of epidemiological indicators or behavioural outcomes are not the most appropriate way of measuring effectiveness in relation to, for example, school based interventions. A cancer education programme in schools may have as its ultimate aim the reduction in morbidity and mortality from cancer, but it wouldn't be useful for school health promotion coordinators and teachers to put this forward as a goal since they will not generally be in a position to measure these outcomes. Further, the education programme in the school, which might highlight the 'benefits' of a particular diet, the risks associated with smoking and high alcohol consumption and the 'efficacy' of screening services may all be to little effect since the causal relationship between many of these factors and cancer is uncertain. School health promotion programmes often ignore other factors that impact on decision-making about behaviour and lifestyle. These decisions are often multi-determined and very difficult to evaluate. A more realistic and meaningful way of evaluating health promotion in schools would be to develop input proxy indicators that measured the inputs into cancer education programmes (e.g. teaching sessions or training of teachers in this area), combined with intermediate proxy indicators that measured impact of programmes (e.g. change in pupil knowledge or positive attitudes to cancer screening). With these input indicators there would be a need to assess policies that supported (or hindered) the cancer education programme (e.g. school meals policies, smoking policies) as part of a broad process evaluation of the programme implementation.

Needs assessment and Delphi

The Healthy Cities movement provides a second example of an innovative approach to evaluation even if the evaluative methodology is not uniform across the whole programme. For example Dam (1996) offers a way of measuring the effectiveness of a research strategy designed to generate immigrant community health action in a city in the Netherlands. Through a variation on the Delphi technique to assess health needs, the researchers and community health workers developed a four stage approach to promoting community action in the area of health that resulted in community involvement and the establishment of a Health Information Centre. The Delphi variation involved including the immigrant community and the community care workers in the development of the design and content of a mental health programme. The design involved three rounds of open discussions about mental health, its determinants, its manifestations and the means of treating it. The discussions were constructed to use not only the knowledge of experts but to include the experiences of immigrants in the community.

The four stage approach linked a traditional epidemiological needs assessment, based on morbidity data but including standard community profiling, with three other non-traditional stages to needs assessment. First, data from semi-structured interviews with community health care workers were collected. This informed the research team about the perceived needs of the immigrant community in relation to mental health care. Second, the next stage involved interviews with non-professional immigrants which helped to construct individual profiles of the values and culture of the community, their expectations and experiences and their use of health care resources. Finally, and in what constituted the fourth stage, the Delphi method variation was involved, in which the first three stages were presented to community focus groups as a starting point for the discussions.

This approach to research provided a basis for process evaluation which proved to be invaluable in the assessment of the programme in terms of how the four stages worked (or didn't) and how the process might be changed in order to produce a better dialogue between care workers and providers and the community they serve.

Storytelling as case study

The technique described above provides an appropriate precursor to the next illustration of a new approach to evaluation which concentrates on process and intermediate indicators. The 'using stories in health promotion practice approach' seems to have been first realised in Canada (Labonte and Feather 1996), although it may have its roots in the oral history tradition of historical narrative data collection. This method of evaluation includes storytelling by sample group, as a critical component of a case study approach. A case approach links together a broad range of views and reflections of a study sample, which may include practitioners, community members and others.

Case story descriptions, analysed and aggregated, may provide a much wider and informed data set than other forms of qualitative research because they can gather information on past events, on individuals in the community, on organisational settings and such like that help us understand why events happened rather than how and when. This form of reflection can help us understand the evaluation process and help to generalise learning into more effective practice.

These three illustrative cases of process evaluation provide some measure of the imaginative use of intermediate indicators that help in the search for realistic and meaningful qualitative effectiveness studies. Many more are provided in this context in subsequent chapters in this book. However if these intermediate or process indicators are to become established and accepted then there is an urgent need to develop a taxonomy or even a hierarchy of qualitative process evaluative methodologies that can rival the quantitative hierarchy that recognises the paramountcy of the randomised control (clinical) trial. Only by doing this can process and intermediate indicators of success survive the rigorous appraisal needed for validity and reliability in the research instrument. Whatever methodology is used the researcher has to be sure that their data is truthful and trustworthy. That is, according to Polit and Hungler (1993), it has demonstrated the four criteria of credibility (confidence in the truth), transferability

(ability to transfer the data to other settings), dependability (the stability of data over time) and confirmability (the neutrality of the data). When a hierarchy is developed that allows these four criteria to be applied rigorously then process and intermediate indicators of success can be considered of 'scientific' merit.

The need to provide appropriate and relevant evidence of success helps in the search for *proof* of effectiveness but it is also an important element in the search for assurance that programmes and other interventions are carried out in the 'best' possible way. This is where the quality assurance (QA) in health promotion helps to provide a framework for ways to *improve* practice.

If a recognised taxonomy or hierarchy for both qualitative and quantitative evaluative methodologies were developed, promoted and used as a quality tool to assist in the assessment of interventions then we would have a form of quality assurance linked to research. However, practitioners also need a form of QA that helps them perform tasks to an agreed best standard in the course of their everyday practice. We would like to discuss QA next by examining its relevance to health promotion practice, by giving an example or two and finally by linking it to effective research.

QUALITY ASSURANCE IN PRACTICE

The current preoccupation with quality assurance is symptomatic of a far wider concern with modern management methods and contemporary management speak and their application to the health care field. This has, in part, been driven by the relatively new competitive and contractual climate in health care delivery and in part by the need to provide effective and efficient services and programmes. Health promotion like other areas of health care has not escaped this influence and has begun to develop ways of approaching quality assurance.

Quality assurance has largely been promoted in health care either through new management arrangements and methods within the process of total quality management or within a clinical setting, through the term audit, particularly clinical audit. However, as Speller *et al.* point out in this volume, the differences are unclear. Indeed the Society of Health Education and Promotion Specialists (SHEPS) in the UK, also refer to audit when discussing QA in health promotion (SHEPS 1992). Certainly the aims of clinical audit, to facilitate continuous quality improvement (CQI), reflect the same aim as total quality management (TQM), to develop a systematic approach to evaluating services and to promote and measure the quality of that service (Ovretveit 1996). These approaches are not dissimilar to the aims of QA in health promotion. In health promotion, practitioners and service providers strive to provide a service based on consumer need that is effective and efficient and is subject to performance measures of some kind (Macdonald 1992).

If there is a form of consensus on what constitutes QA then there is a degree of consensus on the definition of quality itself. Quality in relation to health care provision should provide certain characteristics that reflect the 'needs of the customer' (Sage 1991) 'at the lowest possible cost' (Ovretveit 1996), but 'achieving desirable objectives' (Donabedian 1988). These characteristics of QA in health care provision need then to be applied to the process of the provision itself, to the setting in which the care is provided and to the outcomes of the care.

The needs of the consumer, or in health promotion terms the wider community, is paramount and of primacy in any health promotion programme. It helps determine the focus of work, programme direction and content, but it needs to be balanced by the priorities of the health professional (normally based on epidemiological data) and the cost-effectiveness priorities of managers. The need of the community may be determined in a variety of ways but typically through the judicious use of focus groups using rapid appraisal techniques or through standard questionnaires as assessment instruments. QA can be built into the needs assessment strategy by developing post-intervention methods that rely on, for example, critical incident techniques. This allows members of the community to assess explicitly whether a programme has met and satisfied the identified need. This application of QA to the process of an interventions life has to have standards in order to measure the quality. These standards, which should be quantifiable need to provide a precise indication of consistency. They should initially be based on best existing practice with the cooperation of practitioners, and have a temporal dimension which allows them to improve over time. Standards can be sub-divided into criteria and indicators, depending on how precise the QA process is to be. These two stages, needs assessment and standards setting form the first two parts of the now familiar QA circle (see Figure 1.1).

The set standards are then subject to continual monitoring during the lifetime of the intervention. This monitoring process can be conducted through periodic

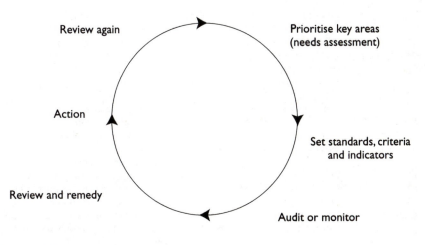

Figure 1.1 Quality assurance circle
Source: Adapted from Ellis and Whittington (1993).

audit of the programme or through other forms of monitoring which might include time and motion studies, observation or other forms of rigorous record keeping, but which allows the 'auditor' to compare practice with the set standards. There may be some controversy about when standards should be set (and by whom). That is, before or after auditing or monitoring (Wilson 1994), but it seems reasonable to set them with the practitioners before a programme is implemented with the proviso that they will be subject to periodic change following audit.

The next stage in the QA circle is designed to determine whether or not the set standards have been reached. If they have been met, then through a further review new standards should be set which demonstrate improvement and the process is repeated. If, however, standards are not met, then the reasons need to be identified. These might be linked to poor initial resources, poor staff training, organisational constraints such as intersectoral working, or even inappropriate audit or monitoring tools. Remedial action is then needed to right the identified causes of not meeting the standards and to bring the health promotion intervention back on course to achieve its aims and to address needs. Quality assurance planning, implementation and review is a critical part of any health promotion programme and should be afforded the same priority as the planning implementation and evaluation of the programme itself. If part of the key areas of work of any health promotion practitioner includes programme planning, management and evaluation, then it is possible to divide the programme into: input; process; output; and outcome. These four stages constitute the totality of an interventions' life, and lend themselves to the application of particular work functions associated with each stage and, in turn, to the application of QA measures as identified in Table 1.1.

Table 1.1 Quality assurance measures for a four-stage health promotion programme

Stage	Work/function	Quality assurance measures
Inputs:	Needs assessment	Focus groups/critical incidence
	Planning framework	Business plan/meetings/targets
	Staff training	Qualifications/experience
	Resource management	Efficiency/effectiveness
Process:	Needs assessment response	Speed/type of response
	Role delineation	Equitable responsibilities
	Operational meetings	Monitoring
		Reports/record keeping
Outputs:	Change/increase in service provision	Change meets consumer needs
	Change in health-related behaviour	Behavioural change supports
	Change in environment	health policy enacted upon
Outcomes:	Better health	Improved morbidity/mortality data
	Sustainable change for health	structural change monitored and evident

Table 1.2 Quality assurance measures for a particular work function

Work/function	Standards	Criteria	Indicators
Planning framework Draft business plan	Planning group constituted and meetings arranged	Group represents all relevant agencies and meets every week	Business plan published on time All agencies and consumers endorse it

Whilst every stage is critical for the successful completion of a programme the crucial first step in the process is the health needs assessment function. All stages and functions will require cooperation from a range of 'consumers', professionals and agencies if the intervention is to be relevant and of high quality. Standards can be applied to every work function and these standards can in turn, be broken down into criteria and indicators as shown in Table 1.2.

QA offers a practical step by step guide to best practice, for health promotion specialists working in the community on a day to day basis and helps them develop a means of assessing and measuring the quality of their work. It is not an exact science however and it still needs further refinement and innovation for the best features of QA to be truly applicable to health promotion. This means that attempts to demonstrate the effectiveness of health promotion and improve its quality are currently limited by the following factors:

- a lack of suitable process evaluation measures or indicators to assess quality appropriate to the needs of health promotion practitioners; and pressure to borrow inappropriate ones from elsewhere;
- the practice of repeating interventions and thereby learning from previous experience seems alien to health promotion;
- little discussion occurs in health promotion journals or communication networks that helps to build a knowledge base – each article or paper is one off with little follow-up or debate;
- there is a dearth of studies on evaluation strategy, including quality measures related to research design. Bias exists towards single effectiveness studies using individual outcome measures, such as knowledge and attitude change, in small groups (based on knowledge/attitude/practice models of traditional health education). Internal validity and reliability are seen as quality controls. There is a lack of work on the effectiveness of broader structural changes in either policy or environment;
- good linkages between research and practice in health promotion are not well established;
- with regard to quality assurance, there is lack of agreement on a framework or common terminology. There is confusion over the use of outcome measures, quality indicators and their inter-relationship;

- there is still a basic lack of understanding regarding the ideology, methods and practice of health promotion;
- these above limitations mean health promotion exists in a culture that encourages reinvention of the wheel, which demonstrates weaknesses in its theoretical and practical foundations.

Therefore, inappropriate traditional approaches to evaluation and quality assurance are currently being forced on health promotion. This is occurring for two basic reasons: first, the dominance of the biomedical outcome model and evidence-based health care (reinforced by demands of managerial/financial control and professional-bias); and second, the lack of appropriate dedicated methods and measurements to evaluate health promotion, as indicated above.

ENABLING AND EMPOWERING: THE FUTURE

In order to *prove* and *improve* health promotion theory and practice the following needs must be met:

- a common framework for assessing the effectiveness and quality of health promotion activities in common with an understanding of the underlying philosophy, values, aims and objectives, and methods and practice (Ziglio 1996);
- a common set of criteria to assess effectiveness and quality (Catford 1993);
- a systematic and rigorous review procedure, using appropriate research methods with common quality criteria, relating together to all components of health promotion action. These methods and criteria will need to be diverse and relate to practical systems and processes, including coordination, within continuous quality improvement (Ovretveit 1996).

These three points need to be supported by a broadly based QA programme. However, the application of QA indicators to health promotion practice and research can seem somewhat mechanistic if confined to the illustrations outlined above. To be truly health promoting we need to struggle with the notion of applying measures to health promotion programmes that are characterised by approaches referred to earlier and reinforced by Dreber (1996), namely enabling and empowering. Therefore health promotion interventions need to take cognisance of the ethical and philosophical roots that support programme planning and implementation. These roots can be summarised in the form of a ten point code that recognises (amongst others), the value of socially just interventions: the application of principles of equity and equality; of needs assessment and participation of communities; of an ethical framework for action; as well as concern for effectiveness, efficiency and the environment. This ten point code has been elaborated on elsewhere (Macdonald 1997) but it is only by *striving to understand* the difficulty in trying to develop appropriate quality indicators and research instruments for these more philosophical dimensions of health promotion interventions, that we begin to address the nub of what constitutes best and effective practice.

References

Allensworth, D. (1994) The Research Base for Innovative Practices in School Health Education at the Secondary Level. *Journal of School Health* 64: 180–187.

Allison, K. and Rootman, I. (1996) Scientific Research and Community Participation in Health Promotion Research: Are They Complete? *Health Promotion International* 11, 4: 333–340.

Baum, F. (1988) Community-based Research for the New Public Health. *Health Promotion International* 3, 3.

Bennett, P. and Murphy, S. (1997) *Psychology and Health Promotion*. Buckingham. Open University Press.

Burrows, R. (1996) Health Promotion and the Vocabulary of the Internal Market. *Health Education Research: Theory and Practice* 11, 3: 365–366.

Caplan, R. (1993) The Importance of Social Theory for Health Promotion: from Description to Reflexivity. *Health Promotion International* 8, 147–157.

Catford, J. (1993) Auditing Health Promotion: What are the Vital Signs? *Health Promotion International* 8, 2: 67–68.

Costongs, C. and Springett, J. (1997) Towards a Framework for the Evaluation of Health-related Policies in Cities. *Evaluation* 3, 3: 3–7.

Dam, J. Ten (1996) Healthy Research in Cities: a Case Study on the Translation of Health Research into Action in the Netherlands. *Health Promotion International* 11, 4: 265–276.

Davies, J.K. and Kelly, M. (eds) (1993) *Healthy Cities: Research and Practice*. London. Routledge.

Donabedian, A. (1988) The Quality of Care: How Can it Be Assessed? *JAMA* 260: 1,743–1,748.

Dreber, A. (1996) How Can We Ensure in Practice that Quality and Effectiveness are Built and Implemented into Health Promotion Interventions. Paper presented at 3rd European Conference on the Effectiveness of Health Promotion and Education. Turin.

Ellis, R. and Whittington, D. (1993) *Quality Assurance in Health Care: a Handbook*. London. Edward Arnold.

Evans, D., Head, M.J. and Speller, V. (1994) *Assuring Quality in Health Promotion: How to Develop Standards of Good Practice*. London. Health Education Council.

Gatherer, A., Parfit, J., Porter, E. and Vessey, M. (1979) *Is Health Education Effective?* Health Education Council Monograph 2. London. Health Education Council.

Green, L. and Lewis, F. (1986) *Measurement and Evaluation in Health Education and Health Promotion*. Palo Alto, Cal. Mayfield Publishing Company.

Health Education Authority (1997) *Summary of Key Findings from the European Network of Health Promoting Schools Survey*, London. HEA.

Hepworth, J. (1997) Evaluation in Health Outcomes Research: Linking Theories, Methodologies and Practice in Health Promotion. *Health Promotion International* 12, 3: 233–238.

Labonte, R. and Feather, J. (1996) *Handbook on Using Stories in Health Promotion Practice*. Canada. Prairie Region Health Promotion Centre.

Lipsey, K., Crosse, S., Drinkle, J. and Stobalt, G. (1985) Evaluation: the State of the Art and the Sorry State of the Science. *New Directions in Programme Evaluation* 27: 7–28.

Macdonald, G. (ed.) (1992) *Quality in Health Promotion*. Cardiff. Health Promotion Wales.

Macdonald, G. (1996) Where Next for evaluation? *Health Promotion International* 11, 3: 171–173.

Macdonald, G. (1997) Quality Indicators and Health Promotion Effectiveness. *Promotion & Education* 4, 2: 5–8.

Macdonald, G. and Bunton, R. (1993) Health Promotion: Discipline or Disciplines? In R. Bunton and G. Macdonald (eds) *Health Promotion: Disciplines and Diversity*. 2nd edn. London. Routledge: 6–19.

Macdonald, G., Veen, C. and Tones, K. (1996) Evidence for Success in Health Promotion: Suggestions for Improvement. *Health Education Research: Theory and Practice* 11, 3: 367–376.

Means, R. and Smith, R. (1988) Implementing a Pluralistic Approach to Evaluation in Health Education. *Policy and Politics* 16: 134–139.

Nutbeam, D. (1996) Achieving Best Practice in Health Promotion: Improving the Fit between Research and Practice. *Health Education Research: Theory and Practice* 11, 3: 317–326.

Nutbeam, D., Smith, C., Murphy, S. and Catford, J. (1993) Maintaining Evaluation Designs in a Long-term Community-based Health Promotion Programme: Heartbeat Wales Case Study. *Journal of Epidemiology and Community Health* 47, 127–133.

Ovretveit, J. (1996) Quality in Health Promotion. *Health Promotion International* 11, 1: 55–62.

Peberdy, A. (1997) Evaluation in Health Promotion: Why Do It? in Katz, J. and Peberdy, A. (eds) *Promoting Health: Knowledge and Practice*. Buckingham. Open University/Macmillan.

Polit, D. and Hungler, B. (1993) *Essentials of Nursing Research*. Philadelphia. Lippincott.

Raeburn, J. (1992) Health Promotion Research with Heart: Keeping a People Perspective. *Canadian Journal of Public Health* 6. Supplement 5: 520–524.

Sage, G. (1991) Customers and the NHS. *International Journal of Health Care Quality Assurance* 4, 3: 16–20.

Sheldon, T., Song, F. and Davey-Smith, G. (1993) *Purchasing and Providing Health Care*. Edinburgh. Churchill Livingstone.

Society of Health Education and Promotion Specialists (1992) *Developing Quality in Health Education and Health Promotion*. SHEPS. GPS. Belfast.

Springett, J. (1998) Quality Measures and Evaluation of Healthy City Policy Initiatives: the Liverpool Experience (this volume).

Whelan, A., Murphy, S. and Smith, C. (1993) *Performance Indicators in Health Promotion: a Review of Possibilities and Problems*. Technical Report No. 2. Cardiff. Health Promotion Wales.

Williams, G. and Popay, J. (1994) Researching the People's Health: Dilemmas and Opportunities for Social Scientists. In Popay, J. and Williams, G. *Researching the People's Health*. London. Routledge.

Wilson, A. (1994) *Changing Practices in Primary Health Care*. London. Health Education Authority.

World Health Organization (1978) *Alma Ata Declaration*. Geneva. WHO.

World Health Organization (1984) *Health Promotion: a Discussion Document on the Concepts and Principles*. Copenhagen. WHO.

World Health Organization (1986) *The Ottawa Charter for Health Promotion*. Copenhagen. WHO.

World Health Organization (1988) *The Adelaide Recommendations*. Geneva. WHO.

World Health Organization (1991) *The Sundsvall Statement on Supportive Environments for Health*. Geneva. WHO.

World Health Organization (1997) *The Jakarta Declaration on Leading Health Promotion into the 21st Century*. Geneva. WHO.

Ziglio, E. (1996) How to Move Forward towards Evidence-based Health Promotion Interventions. Paper presented at 3rd European Conference on the Effectiveness of Health Promotion and Health Education. Turin.

Part 1

Methods for assessing evidence and effectiveness

Chapter 2

Reviewing the evidence for health promotion in the United States[1]

Noreen M. Clark and Kenneth R. McLeroy

BACKGROUND

We have approached this discussion of the knowledge base for health promotion in the United States by addressing three questions. First, what is the context in the country that gives rise to and shapes health promotion efforts? Second, what do we know about health promotion interventions? For example, how effective are various theoretical frameworks and principles that guide practice? Where can programmes be effectively deployed? Which intervention strategies and evaluation methods work best? What are the issues when working with special populations? Third, what models and conceptual approaches will shape health promotion in the future and serve as a basis for assessing quality and effectiveness?

Historical issues

Largely as a result of changes in living conditions and basic public health measures, there has been a dramatic increase in longevity since the start of the twentieth century. In 1900, for example, 4.1 per cent of Americans were over the age of 65. By the end of the century, however, the proportion of the population over the age of 65 increased to an estimated 13 per cent. As the prevalence of chronic conditions is associated with age, the growing number of elderly in the population has had a significant effect on the demand for health care. In 1985, 80 per cent of those over the age of 65 reported one or more chronic condition, 39 per cent reported limitations in their ability to perform routine daily activities, and 22 per cent reported limitations in major activities, such as working, keeping house, or living independently (German and Fried, 1989).

Health care expenditures have increased from 3.5 per cent of all goods and services produced in the United States in 1929 to 11.1 per cent in 1987 (NCHS, 1990), in large part a result of chronic disease. In 1993, the most recent year for which information is available, health care expenditures accounted for 13 per cent of the gross national product. This is a rate of expenditures for health care about 30 per cent higher than in most developed countries.

Primarily to control expenditures, federal, state, and local governments increasingly have focused on prevention. The belief that health promotion and disease prevention may reduce health care costs is drawn from two lines of evidence. The first is studies linking behaviour to health outcomes. The second comprises evaluation reports showing relationships between public health interventions and reduced morbidity and mortality.

Prevention of chronic disease in the United States has generally been focused on behavioural risk factors (see, for example, US Surgeon General's Report on Health Promotion and Disease Prevention, 1979). More recent attention has been paid to the relative contribution of behaviour to premature mortality (McGinnis and Foege, 1993). Despite substantial evidence linking social factors (race, gender, and ethnic discrimination, political disenfranchisement, and poverty) to the aetiology and evolution of chronic diseases (Mechanic 1989), relatively little attention, as yet, has been paid to ameliorating these factors as they directly affect health behaviour or health status.

Good evidence is also available to demonstrate that modifying behaviours may reduce the burden of mortality in the US population. For example, since the 1960s, societal efforts to reduce smoking rates have resulted in less tobacco use in the population, and substantial declines in heart disease and stroke mortality (US Surgeon General, 1989).

CURRENT CONTEXT OF HEALTH PROMOTION AND DISEASE PREVENTION IN THE UNITED STATES

Other contemporary factors are affecting health promotion in the United States. First, is the emergence of managed care systems intended to function as a control on health care expenditures. Unlike most developed countries, the United States has no comprehensive system for assuring or providing universal health care. Rather, health services are provided primarily by individual, group, or corporate practice physicians reimbursed on a fee-for-service basis. With the failure of US health care reform in 1993–94, there has been a desire to constrain health care costs. Managed care plans reimburse clinical services obtained by their enrolled populations on a capitated, rather than a fee-for-service-basis. The financial benefits of keeping a population well are significant and this fact has increased the potential for renewed emphasis on reconfiguring services into managed care plans, primarily from a desired provision of both primary and secondary prevention services by these systems.

Accompanying the emphasis on managed care in the United States are efforts to strengthen the core public health functions. In 1988, the Institute of Medicine (IOM) convened an expert panel to review the extant public health infrastructure, outcomes, and processes. The result was a report on the *Future of Public Health* that continues to have a substantial impact on local, state, and Federal initiatives. In their report, the IOM (1988) identified three core functions of public health: assessment; policy development; and assurance. These functions include ten essential services identified by the Core Public Health Functions Steering Committee of the US Department of Health and Human Services (Lee and Paxman, 1997). Invigorating public health agencies will require a higher level of spending on health promotion and disease prevention activities. Less than 1 per cent of the total expenditures for health care in the United States (Lee *et al.*, 1996) is directed towards prevention. Whether a shift of resources will follow the apparent shift of interest away from curative towards preventive services remains to be seen.

A third contemporary factor affecting health promotion in the United States is the growing evidence, generated through outcome research, of the efficacy of social and behavioural interventions in public health. While many intervention projects, particularly small scale, local ones, are initiated with no or inadequate evaluation designs, funding agencies have increasingly demanded formal evaluations as part of research contracts and grant awards. The extant research on public health interventions in the United States has touched areas as distinct as, for example, clinical interventions for smoking cessation in pregnant women, to formation of community coalitions. The available literature has been used to enhance practice guidelines for preventive services in clinical settings. Current efforts are underway at the Centers for Disease Control and Prevention to develop practice guidelines for community-based programmes based on evaluated interventions.

Yet another factor influencing health promotion in the US is renewed public and professional attention to community culture, interests, and priorities in public health practice. Some funding agencies now routinely require community involvement in intervention efforts, often including the establishment of community coalitions or task forces as a condition for grant funding (McLeroy *et al.*, 1994). Since an adequate level of community capacity may be a necessary condition for programs to be successful, there has been increased interest in developing methods for assessing capacity. The recognition of the reciprocal relationship of individual and collective health has led to interest in determining the impact of health promotion programs on broader aspects of community life.

A final factor in influencing health promotion is the involvement of new providers of service. While the bulk of prevention efforts have traditionally been implemented by government and voluntary health agencies, there are new players on the field. As noted, some managed care plans recognize a connection between health promotion and patient satisfaction, reduced costs, and/or improved health status. As a result, several are experimenting with health promotion interventions that reach beyond clinical settings. In a few cases, regulatory agencies have required that such organizations provide community-wide activities and otherwise support public health efforts. In addition to managed care systems, a variety of for-profit and not-for-profit organizations have increased their involvement in health promotion, including universities, public schools, pharmacies, hospitals, and corporations. As with managed care organizations, the future participation of such entities in health promotion is not assured, but they may comprise important means for reaching selected populations.

WHAT WE KNOW ABOUT HEALTH PROMOTION: INTERVENTION STRATEGIES

It is an oversimplification to say that research undertaken since the 1970s in the US, both to describe and to enhance health promotion, can be easily classified. Nonetheless, we have organized recent work into one of three categories, by virtue of the theoretical principles espoused and methods employed. These categories (discussed in greater length in the last part of this chapter) comprise social behavioural approaches, social ecology, and empowerment. Before considering the similarities and differences in categories of health promotion research undertaken in the recent past, we will provide a status report on findings that cut across the three categories and present results according to the level or scope of the intervention (individual change or community change or change in larger populations reached via mass media); the special population targeted; or the educational or behavioural theory explored. In this discussion we will focus more on interventions that are essentially educational and behavioural in nature than on those that are legislative and administrative. The latter are often potent ways to effect individual and social change, yet the process of achieving new policies and laws is often difficult to describe accurately and outcomes of such interventions are hard to quantify. Therefore, they are less likely to be researched and reported in the literature. Our aim is to present the case for interventions that have received empirical assessment and this goal will naturally cause educational and behavioural approaches to dominate.

It is generally accepted that health problems and interventions to address them must be conceived of comprehensively. That is, we must identify those aspects of a problem that are manifest in individual behaviour, in the social and physical environment of the community, and in the policies regulating both. Interventions aimed at any one of these three levels (individual, community, policy) will affect and be affected by the others. Mass media, which appear to exert powerful influence across the three levels are technologies about which we know surprisingly little.

INDIVIDUAL BEHAVIOUR AND SETTINGS FOR INTERVENTIONS

Most intervention research in health promotion in the US including health education has been directed towards individual behaviour. Since the 1980s a large number of studies has provided evidence that changes in behaviour and improved health status can be realized. Findings from well designed studies have demonstrated, for example, that pre-operative instruction can influence recovery (Daltroy *et al.*, 1989), that education engenders improved compliance (Morisky *et al.*, 1990), disease self-management (Bartholomew *et al.*, 1991), patient–provider communication (Strecher, 1982), use of health services (Clark *et al.*, 1986), symptom profiles and functioning in chronic disease (Clark *et al.*, 1986; Lorig *et al.*, 1985), diet (Winett *et al.*, 1989), exercise level (Mittlemark *et al.*, 1993), and intentions not to smoke (Pierce *et al.*, 1992).

Several generalizations can be made about the work regarding individual behaviour undertaken to date. One is that most successful strategies have been derived from theories of behaviour (Freudenberg *et al.*, 1995). Another is that when viewed in total, that is, all interventions related to a given health problem versus only those meeting some criterion of quality, changes in knowledge exceed changes in behaviour (Lorig *et al.*, 1987; Mullen *et al.*, 1987). Still another is that intervention strategies have been eclectic, employing a range of techniques and theoretical principles (Kovar *et al.*, 1992).

At least two needs are evident given these observations. First, criteria are required to ensure quality in designing interventions. We have to assess existing work to determine the theoretical approaches and principles that have yielded empirical results, consider them a minimum standard, and test them further. One application is not enough to prove a strategy's worth. Second, we need sustained work related to a given health problem. Conducting only a few studies in any one area (e.g., physical functioning, diet) is insufficient to determine the effectiveness of an intervention model.

Settings where health promotion activities are implemented are channels for reaching defined populations (Mullen *et al.*, 1995). The settings most often selected for interventions, schools, worksites, and medical care facilities, also offer the potential for institutionalizing effective interventions through their organizational policies and resource allocations. The setting for some well known health education interventions have been the entire community, for example, to reduce cardiovascular risk behaviour. Some have enjoyed a degree of success (Farquhar *et al.*, 1977), others have not (Luepker *et al.*, 1994). But far and away, the greatest number of rigorously evaluated health education interventions for changing individual behaviour have been conducted in specific institutional settings.

SCHOOLS

In an era more oriented towards prevention of disease, earlier intervention will probably become a goal to obviate, as soon as possible, diseases that are costly in both human and economic terms. Reaching children will become even more important and schools a more significant venue, and there are strong precedents for work in this area (Mullen *et al.*, 1995).

School health education curricula for middle school children have influenced their knowledge, attitudes, and behaviour regarding risk reduction (Christenson *et al.*, 1985) although not all programs can claim success (Ross *et al.*, 1991). Secondary school students participating in health education curricula have decreased their alcohol, tobacco, and drug use, but not seat belt use behaviour (Ross *et al.*, 1991). They have improved their diets (Walter and Wynder, 1989) and delayed sexual activity or used a condom when engaging in sex (Kirby *et al.*, 1994). Many children in the United States have chronic disease. At least one study suggests that self-management education provided at the school site can improve the health status and school performance of children with asthma (Evans *et al.*, 1987).

These findings give rise to other issues. What are the behaviours best addressed in school programmes? Is the best way to intervene through traditional curricular approaches? What are the appropriate interventions for which age groups? How much education is needed to sustain change over time and have an effect in adulthood? The potential for school as the setting for health promotion has not yet been adequately mined.

WORKSITE

Reaching the population through worksite programs has tremendous appeal as most US citizens of working age are employed. Work-based programs directed towards cardiovascular risk reduction, diet, back injury, arthritis self-management, have shown small but significant effects on participants' behaviour (Pelletier, 1993). They have also been shown to generate savings equivalent to their costs. But, many questions need answering if we intend to maximize the potential for work-based programmes. Between one-quarter to one-half of those given the opportunity actually participate (Glasgow *et al.*, 1993). What groups are best reached at work? What are alternative ways to reach them? How can health promotion be integrated to be more seamless in the work day? What policies and aspects of the social environment influence behaviour change? Which programs are simultaneously most effective and most affordable?

HEALTH CARE SETTINGS

It is in the medical care setting that the bulk of rigorously evaluated secondary prevention intervention studies have been carried out in the United States. Most have concerned chronic disease and have been mounted in concert with or assuming the existence of clinical services. Secondary prevention may become a growth industry as the United States health care system develops a prevention focus. Clinical outcome, quality of care, patient satisfaction, and disease management, including health education, are being closely scrutinized by managed care, health maintenance, and other organizations redrawing the services picture. There is evidence to suggest the scrutiny is warranted and these interventions make a difference. Changed patient behaviour and/or health status has been associated with programs provided in conjunction with clinical services for asthma (Wigal *et al.*, 1990), arthritis (Lorig *et al.*, 1987), coronary artery disease (Mullen *et al.*, 1992), diabetes (Padgett *et al.*, 1988). Positive change related to non-chronic conditions have also been documented, for example, reduced pain (Jones, 1986) and improved pregnancy outcomes. Computer-based interventions to further clinical goals have shown promise. For example, to decrease smoking (Strecher *et al.*, 1994) and motivate women to seek mammography (Skinner *et al.*, 1993).

Still, many questions remain. What elements of an intervention must be in place to achieve quality of life and clinical goals related to specific diseases? Which approaches for which conditions are linked to outcomes? How can problems be overcome related to time and cost of programs and ability of health care professionals to successfully educate their patients? Training professionals is a promising route to reaching more patients and influencing their behaviour (Hollis *et al.*, 1993), but to date few programs (Inui *et al.*, 1976) have demonstrated change for patients as a result of training health professionals. The existing work in health care settings provides a strong basis for future research. The population with chronic disease is increasing, and the need to achieve clinical and other outcomes related to patient functioning is increasingly critical. Research related to interventions in health care settings continues to be a compelling line of inquiry.

The next level of research across these diverse settings for health promotion may concern how to get effective programs adopted. We have achieved successes, yet these have not been widely replicated. How can model programs best be disseminated? There are some good examples of program dissemination (Gottlieb *et al.*, 1994; Stone *et al.*, 1994). What can we learn from these examples?

COMMUNITY LEVEL INTERVENTIONS

It has been argued (IOM, 1988) that approaches focused on individual behaviour leave out important influences in the social and cultural environment. To be effective, interventions must have an impact on social norms and accepted ways of functioning that may be deleterious to health. Further, this influence must be of a type that is acceptable to communities of people, that is, consistent with their values and their definitions of health and quality of life. Several community focused strategies have been examined in the US since the late 1980s that attempt to connect health professionals to communities, provide access to services, and develop community capacity to recognize and resolve health problems. Successful strategies have involved social networks (Gottlieb, 1985) and lay health advisors, natural helpers in a community who have the stature and ability to reach others (Eng and Young, 1992; Watkins *et al.*, 1994). Forming coalitions of key community groups and organizations has also been shown to increase people's participation in health programs (Flynn, 1992) and mobilize community residents to take specific actions related to health (Rivo *et al.*, 1992).

Strategies to imbue community residents with a sense of efficacy and capacity, often referred to as empowerment strategies, have been shown to contribute positively to health objectives: for example, improved birth outcomes for homeless women (Overbo *et al.*, 1994), change in government health policy (Wang and Burris, 1994), and in increased public awareness, for example, of the consequences of excess drinking (Wallerstein and Bernstein, 1988). Few rigorous studies of interventions focused on community-wide change are available, and this seems a very promising area of work. The research design and measurement issues are significant in this form of research (Israel *et al.*, 1995). Our evaluation methods are not yet a match for the complexity of the interventions. Further, community-wide interventions often aim at intermediate outcomes, say, forming coalitions or increasing a sense of empowerment, and the link from these to improvements in health have not been examined. The potential for community targeted approaches to reach large numbers of people, especially populations that have been underserved makes them very appealing and worthy of much more attention than they receive.

POLICY LEVEL INTERVENTIONS

Policy research related to health promotion is essentially of two types, organizational policy and public policy affecting large numbers of citizens. Concerning the first type, Mullen *et al.* (1995) suggest that several studies regarding workplace smoking show that achieving compliance with policies within organizations is not easy (Rigotti *et al.*, 1994). Studies also show that efforts to establish worksite no smoking policies are related to the strength of local smoking ordinances (Pierce *et al.*, 1994). Studies comparing the effectiveness of worksite smoking bans compared to policies restricting, but not prohibiting, smoking find that bans are easier to enforce (Borland *et al.*, 1992; Gottlieb *et al.*, 1992) and achieve success in eliminating environmental tobacco smoke. Mullen *et al.* (1995) note that such policies can reduce the amount of smoking by employees although prevalence of smoking depends on several factors, including the nature of the worksite policy (Borland *et al.*, 1991; Rosenstock *et al.*, 1986; Sorensen *et al.*, 1992).

Public policy interventions (Steckler *et al.*, 1995) refer to efforts to bring about new laws or administrative regulations that intend to change the physical or social environment to be more protective of health. All states in the US have laws prohibiting the sale of cigarettes to persons under 18 or 19 years of age. Nationwide, however, Brownson *et al.* (1995) note that three out of four tobacco retailers sell illegally to children (Cummings *et al.*, 1994; DiFranza *et al.*, 1987; US Dept of Health and Human Services, 1994). Further, when minors try to purchase cigarettes out of vending machines, they are successful 88 per cent of the time (Pierce *et al.*, 1992; US Dept of Health and Human Services, 1994). Data from one study in the states of Illinois and Massachusetts suggest that stringent enforcement of youth access laws results in lower smoking prevalence in adolescents (DiFranza *et al.*, 1992; Jason *et al.*, 1991). One study suggests that not all the means of restricting access work effectively. Forster *et al.* (1992) showed that a city ordinance requiring vending machines to be fitted with electronic locking devices to prevent access to underage smokers was an unsuccessful policy with over one-third of merchants failing to comply with the ordinance within three months of its establishment.

Excise taxing is another public policy approach assessed in recent studies. Data suggest rises in the cost of cigarettes of 10 per cent can result in a 4 per cent drop in prevalence of adult smoking (National Cancer Institute, 1993; US Dept of Health and Human Services, 1992; Warner, 1986). Other public policy interventions have been shown to be successful in protecting worksites from toxins (Dept of Labor, 1980), eliminating toxic substances from transport through neighbourhoods (Freudenberg, 1984), and setting aside smoke-free public places (Bierer and Rigotti, 1992) to name a few.

Interventions to engender policy change may be among the most compelling (Steckler *et al.*, 1995) as the possibilities for influencing the behaviour of large numbers of people are great. To date we have few evaluation precedents to serve as a guide. The evaluation problems are tricky to solve. Ideally, assessment would demonstrate that the intervention strategy produced the policy change, the policy change produced the desired behaviour and the behaviour contributed to the health outcome. Making these connections clear cut may be impossible. The challenge may be to identify indicators that most would accept as reliable and valid signs that change is occurring in the desired direction. Difficulties notwithstanding, the potential payoff associated with policy directed interventions probably offsets the costs of learning how we can assess their success.

MASS COMMUNICATIONS

Conventional wisdom and very few studies tell us that mass media can create awareness of health problems (Rice and Atkin, 1990), and influence perceptions about health (Wallack, 1990), and even change health behaviour (Montgomery, 1993). The media are thought to exert significant influence on individual behaviour, community environments, and development of policy (Steckler *et al.*, 1995). It has been suggested that three forms of media-related interventions deserve study: public health campaigns; media advocacy, that is influencing media to examine a given health-related problem; and enter-education, that is, promoting healthful practices by inserting information and role models into media entertainment formats (television, computer and video games, and the like). Undertaking evaluation of these forms of intervention requires new research designs, methods, and measures. But, given the boom in media-related technology and informatics, the potential for such strategies to shape health behaviour and influence health status could increase exponentially in the next two decades.

WORK WITH UNDERSERVED POPULATIONS

Issues arise regarding health promotion for special population groups: groups of similar culture, gender, age. In the United States, the official classifications we employ (African American, Native American), and the less official terms we use (e.g., elderly, adolescent) to describe these populations often have very little meaning either to health professionals or to the people so labelled (Marin et al., 1995). We have had the tendency to view groups of people that share some characteristic (e.g., race, language, country of origin) as being of the same culture. This is far from accurate. The cultures represented within any broad category of people (e.g., Asian Americans, elderly) are very diverse.

The idea of long standing, that there is an 'average person' in the United States, has been influenced by existing data which don't account for large and growing segments of our population. Interventions based on these data and developed for general audiences of 'average Americans' are probably much less effective than those which take into account the culture, social norms, and traditional practices of subgroups of the population. While some data exist to support this observation (Perez-Stable et al., 1993; Rogers, 1993; Uba, 1992), we need more comparative research to demonstrate what we all suspect to be the case; group specific programs are more effective. But, further, we need to understand how and why they are more effective.

Research evaluating the relative advantages of interventions designed for diverse groups is very limited but some data describing psychosocial factors and health practices clearly indicate group differences. For example, recent work in HIV/AIDS prevention has illustrated significant cultural differences in condom use (Gielen et al., 1994; Rosser 1991). Motives for smoking and using alcohol appear to differ by ethnic group (Marin et al., 1989; Marin et al., 1993). Self-management of disease seems to differ (Clark et al., 1990), as does blood pressure control (Whelton et al., 1992), diet and exercise (Cohen et al., 1993), and so on. But we don't know what gives rise to these differences and what kinds of intervention best account for them.

Preliminary evaluative work suggests that some health promotion approaches may be better than others in reaching diverse, underserved populations. Some have been linked to changed health behaviour or health status. Peer counselling, for example, has been shown to be effective with older adults with arthritis (Lorig and Gonzalez, 1992), with African American women at risk of AIDS (Gielen *et al.*, 1994), in smoking cessation with Latino groups (Perez-Stable *et al.*, 1993). Focusing on family members as educators and caregivers appears to produce results with older adults with debilitating disease (Connell *et al.*, 1992), and among groups of Native Americans (Burhansstipanov and Dresser, 1993). Self-help groups, church leaders as educators, training of lay health advisors, all these approaches seem to hold promise (Eng, 1993; Perez-Stable *et al.*, 1993; Stillman *et al.*, 1993; Watkins *et al.*, 1994).

Effective ways to work in diverse cultures have to be empirically derived, and may even require new theories of behaviour. We need data that describe how culturally relevant and appropriate approaches work, and data that illustrate the relative benefits of taking one approach rather than another. We have to be much more creative in designing interventions to build on traditional practices, and cultural norms. We have to use evaluative methods that ensure a fair test of these new approaches (Israel *et al.*, 1995). Part of the evaluative process includes coming to understand how different groups of people define functioning, quality of life, and health, and take measurements accordingly (Eng and Parker, 1994). The impact and outcome measures we conventionally use to assess interventions may need to be adapted or replaced in light of people's diverse expectations and values. The extent to which interventions are able to prevent disease or reduce the disability, disruption, and cost it generates in the society as a whole, may be directly related to how closely they address the unique experience of diverse subgroups of the population.

THEORIES UNDERLYING HEALTH PROMOTION EFFORTS

The period since the 1970s has been rich in theoretical and empirical work related to health promotion (Freudenberg *et al.*, 1995). We have at our disposal a range of excellent theoretical constructs to guide research and practice. But there is always some confusion in the way the word theory is used by researchers and practitioners. For sake of discussion, we will present theories popular in US health promotion efforts according to their utility as follows: (1) those predicting or explaining behaviour; (2) conceptual frameworks for practice; (3) theoretical principles.

The first type of theory attempts to predict or explain why people behave as they do, related to their health. These may be theories that focus primarily on psychological factors such as the Health Belief Model (Janz and Becker, 1984), Health Locus of Control (Wallston and Wallston, 1978), Attribution Theory (Lewis and Daltroy, 1990), the theory of Reasoned Action (Ajzen and Fishbein, 1980), the Transtheoretical Model (Stages of Change) (Prochaska and DiClemente, 1986). Or, they may address the interaction of psychological and social environmental factors such as social cognitive theory (Parcel *et al.*, 1990), self-regulation (Clark and Zimmerman, 1990), Freire's psychosocial model (Freire, 1973), theories of social support and social networks (Stewart, 1989).

There is also an important type of theory that is essentially a framework for practice. These are theories that describe the systemic, structural, or political conditions under which interventions can be made to be effective and efficacious. Theories, particularly relevant to health promotion, include, for example, Precede/Proceed (Green and Kreuter, 1991), PATCH (Simons-Morton *et al.*, 1988), the social ecological model (Hancock, 1993; McLeroy *et al.*, 1988; Stokols, 1992), and the growing body of work on empowerment (Special Issue, HEQ, 1994a, 1994b). There are also a number of theoretical principles that have evolved from predictive and explanatory theories and conceptual frameworks for practice and have been associated with evidence that health status and/or behaviour change have occurred. These include, for example, the principle of tailoring advice and health messages (Freudenberg and Zimmerman, 1995), contracting (Janz *et al.*, 1984), and various communication techniques (Becker, Maiman, 1980; Clark *et al.*, 1994a).

There is, however, somewhat limited empirical evidence about how these theories work in whole and/or part. That is not to say that they have not received or are currently garnering a fair amount of attention in the US. Nonetheless, we are still at a rudimentary stage of understanding: (1) how they actually function to produce results; (2) if some are better than others in producing outcomes; (3) which components or critical mass of constituent concepts or principles is needed to achieve change; and (4) which are more or less relevant to different problems and populations of potential learners.

There are only a few cases, for example, Health Locus of Control (Wallston and Wallston, 1978) and the Transtheoretical Model (Prochaska and DiClemente, 1986), where significant effort has gone into developing measures sensitive to change and applicable to a variety of health promotion problems. But even in cases where this type of effort has been expended, constructs and scales have not been widely or diversely validated.

There is the related though the somewhat different problem of how to adequately apply theoretical constructs in an intervention so that effects may be evaluated. Some theories are easier to apply than others. Social cognitive theory (Parcel *et al.*, 1990), for example, aims to explain how health behaviour comes about. Designing interventions based on these explanations is somewhat evident. However, other theories, for example the Health Belief Model (Janz and Becker, 1984), aim only to *predict* behaviour and provide very little to indicate how the factors influencing it can be manipulated. Knowing that when one believes the consequences of his smoking are serious he is more likely to quit does not inherently explain *how* to make him believe in the seriousness. Because translation of theory to 'real life' is not always easy, interventions have not always comprised strong applications. They have also tended to be eclectic, drawing bits and pieces from a variety of available constructs, that is, they are not purely one theory or another. Perhaps as a result, we have not progressed as much as we might wish in identifying how theories work, and which are most robust and valuable in achieving change.

Assessing the contribution of conceptual frameworks for practice, poses additional problems. One is that these frameworks combine not only what we know about human behaviour and influences in the social environment but also what we wish the ideal situation to be. Practice in a democratic society reflects what we value. Empowerment theories (Special Issue HEQ, 1994a, 1994b), for example, are based on the belief that equality and equity of participation are related to access to needed health services and physical and mental health status. But they are also based on the idea that participation is a right of citizenship. Perhaps the most widely used practice model is Precede/ Proceed (Green and Kreuter, 1991) and one reason may be that it values efficient as well as effective use of resources, a tenet important in equitable delivery of public health services. The point is that practice models do not purport to explain or predict behaviour. Rather, they describe the individual, organizational, and community-wide conditions, processes, and values that should be fostered to bring about change.

Another dilemma in determining the relative merit of different conceptual frameworks for research and practice rests in the fact that they are so comprehensive. They often try to account for the potential learner and range of factors influencing his or her health behaviour, the health professional and the diverse influences on his or her performance, the participating organizations and the spectrum of organizational factors enabling and detracting from the implementation of the intervention, the norms, beliefs, cultural patterns and economic factors evident in the community where the education takes place, and so on. The comprehensive nature of such theory gives rise to several questions: (1) How does one ascertain that the model has been adequately applied? (2) Can models of practice be tested in the same way we test theories of behaviour? (3) Do all the wide-ranging elements need to be in place for a model to receive a fair evaluation? (4) How are changes attributable to a given practice model to be separated from those attributable to the behavioural theories also employed? (5) What are the appropriate outcomes for assessing conceptual frameworks as applied in practice? They appear to differ from those appropriate for behavioural theories. For example, is a reasonable test of a model drawn from social ecological theory institutionalization of a program regardless of whether or not the health behaviour of the program target audience changed?

To make matters more complex, both behavioural theories and conceptual frameworks for practice give rise to theoretical principles. The fact is, some approaches to behaviour change and professional practice are known to achieve certain ends. If individuals have influence in decision-making they appear to be more satisfied with the decision (Israel and Schuman, 1990). If people make public their intention to change, for example to follow a low fat diet, they are more likely to do so (Janz *et al.*, 1984). But these principles, important as they may be, provide only a glimpse at behaviour change and professional practice. They may be important, even necessary, in interventions but they do not appear to be sufficient to describe the mechanisms of change related to complex health problems. And, as is true with the other two categories of theory, the extent to which they produce extensive or long-lasting results or prove effective with diverse populations hasn't been demonstrated. The richness in the range of theories available for designing and evaluating health promoting interventions gives rise to difficult questions and dilemmas.

QUANTITATIVE AND QUALITATIVE APPROACHES TO EVALUATION BASED ON THESE CONCEPTS

What is needed so that our evaluation designs, methods, and measures are employed most effectively in pursuit of public health? The social and behavioural sciences have borrowed heavily from the physical sciences, employing, primarily, experimental research designs and quantitative methods. Quasi-experimental evaluation designs (Clark *et al.*, 1986; Clark *et al.*, 1992; Clark *et al.*, 1994b; COMMIT Research Group, 1991; Cook and Campbell, 1979; Dignan *et al.*, 1991; Hanson and Graham, 1991; Michielutte *et al.*, 1989) have been developed in the attempt to achieve a comparable level of laboratory control in the natural settings where most health promotion researchers work. These designs and methods are an effort to account for all the influences that might produce a result instead of, or in addition to, the intervention. They are considered the most credible precisely because they have been successfully used in biomedical research. However, in the transition from that venue to evaluation of health promotion initiatives, the designs may have lost some of their robustness given the number of uncontrollable factors at play in virtually all contexts in which these interventions are delivered. Few provide all the information that we need when assessing interventions that are essentially social, psychological, and behavioural in their construction and intention.

It has been noted (Israel *et al.*, 1995) that while collecting quantitative data gives us an idea of the dimension of effects and enables us to identify salient relationships among and between variables of interest, these data may oversimplify complex facets of a problem and fail to convey fully the richness and texture of human experience. Collection and analyses of qualitative data to complement quantitative approaches in health related evaluation are becoming not only accepted but popular (Basch, 1987; Israel *et al.*, 1994; Mullen *et al.*, 1986; Steckler, 1989). In being 'qualitative' researchers have borrowed from work in anthropology and other fields where ethnographic methods are used to describe the subtleties and nuances of culture. Ways to more effectively bring together both approaches are needed (Israel *et al.*, 1995). For some, the terms 'quantitative' and 'qualitative' suggest that evaluation is a bifurcated process rather than different elements of the same process. Ideally, most evaluations would include sufficient quantitative data to assess the reach and generalizability of an intervention, and qualitative data to determine the depth and significance of change for individuals and communities (including unintended effects, if any).

What is the right balance or mix of methods to provide the richest evaluative picture? What designs and methods are most appropriate for which problems and populations? The heterogeneity of society and the complexity of health problems and solutions likely demand a variety of approaches to evaluation. No one way applies to all situations. To date confidence has been greatest in quantitative, experimental approaches. We need to develop ways to make these approaches better fit the type of problems we are studying. We also need to explore the potential for qualitative approaches; determine how they round out or change the evaluative picture. We need to recognize and employ existing valid and reliable qualitative methods, and develop new ones that will generate as much confidence as conventional quantitative ones. We need to discover how the two ways of thinking about evaluation can be integrated most successfully in assessments of interventions. This integration, of course, would include enhanced use of statistical analyses.

FUTURE DIRECTIONS

Conceptual frameworks for health promotion/disease prevention research and practice in the United States

Increasingly, philosophies of science emphasize the *interrelationships* among theory, research questions, research methods, research findings, and interpretations of the results. It is important, in this regard, to recognize that much of the research and practice in health promotion and disease prevention in the United States has been guided by a social-behavioural orientation that has not emphasized context and relationships. Thus, health promotion and disease interventions have focused on changing the knowledge, attitudes, skills and behaviours of individuals in given populations through the application of methods drawn primarily from the social and behavioural sciences, often social psychology (McLeroy *et al.*, 1988; Guttman, unpublished; Stokols, 1996). Moreover, program evaluations have historically emphasized experimental research design, statistical methods, and inference.

A result of the social behavioural focus in health promotion and disease prevention in the United States is a dearth of knowledge on a more comprehensive range of issues that probably affect our ability to improve the health of populations, including:

- the importance of program context – such as setting, community characteristics, characteristics of the target population, etc. – program design,
  implementation and outcomes (Mullen *et al.*, 1995);
- the role of cultural and social factors, particularly in economically disadvantaged and minority groups, that mediate the effects of program interventions on outcomes (McLeroy *et al.*, 1995);
- how to tailor programs for disadvantaged and disenfranchised populations
  (Marin *et al.*,1995);
- the relative effectiveness of behavioural interventions and strategies to
  change the social environment, such as formal and informal social networks, organizations, the physical environment, and culture (Steckler *et
  al.*, 1995);
- evaluation strategies for assessing changes in program context or system-
  wide properties (Israel *et al.*, 1995);
- the relative efficacy and effectiveness of newer theories and their practice-
  related principles (Freudenberg *et al.*, 1995).

There are competing conceptual frameworks to the dominant social and behavioural approach to health promotion emerging in the United States
(McLeroy *et al.*, 1988; Winett *et al.*, 1989; Stokols, 1996; Wallerstein and
Bernstein, 1994; Fetterman *et al.*, 1996). For the purposes of this discussion,
to draw attention to some essential differences in how current approaches are
conceptualized and tested, we have organized these (risking great oversimplification) into three categories. Table 2.1 summarizes basic tenets of approaches
falling into these categories and compares the dominant social-behavioural
perspective with two emerging ones, social ecology and empowerment. The
table contrasts the three approaches along a number of dimensions, including
the primary audience for the intervention, philosophy or goals, intervention
methods, preferred research and evaluation methods, anticipated outcomes,
and the primary audience for the research findings.[2]

As suggested in Table 2.1, the primary goal in social-behavioural approaches
is behavioural change (group or individual) and related changes in health
status or health conditions. By contrast, social ecological approaches focus on
changes in the social environment, including subsystems, such as the interpersonal
environment (families, social networks), organizations (schools, workplaces,
etc.), community (e.g., inter-organizational relationships), culture, the physical
environment, etc. Empowerment approaches emphasize developing capacity
of individuals and communities to change the social context or conditions
that constrain their health, particularly through altering power relationships
within and among enfranchised and disenfranchised groups. Intervention strategies
used in the social-behavioural approach must largely be inferred from behavioural
science theories since, as noted, few contain explicit directions on how to
produce change. Intervention methods within a social ecology framework are
similarly inferred but draw more fully on systems theories and models and

Table 2.1 Comparative frameworks for health promotion and disease prevention approaches

Paradigm or framework	Target of intervention	Philosophy or goals	Intervention methods	Research and evaluation methods	Acceptable outcomes	Primary audience for research findings
Social behavioural	Individuals Groups Community organizations Populations	Change behaviour however defined Change health status or conditions relevant to health status	Theory-based, largely drawn from social behavioural theories Focused on individual or group behaviour	Emphasis on experimental or quasi-experimental designs	Evidence of behavioural change and changes in related health problems, conditions, or concerns	Researchers, political decision-makers
Social ecological	Systems	Subsystems are embedded within larger systems Change political, economic, social, physical systems Changing subsystems changes behaviours, and changes subsystems	Theory-based, but emphasizes systems theory Multiple levels of theories and interventions	Emphasis on combining qualitative and quantitative approaches Application of traditional methods and designs to assess system changes	Evidence of change in subsystems or systems	Researchers, political decision-makers
Empowerment	Individuals Groups Communities	Change power relationships Change the social context or conditions	Emphasis on participatory approaches Value on reflective dialogue and action	Emphasis on qualitative approaches Value on participatory evaluation	Process indicators Evidence of changes in power relations in individuals, groups or communities	Participants in the process, other stakeholders

emphasize systems change at multiple levels of a society. Empowerment approaches emphasize participatory processes and reflective action by individuals and communities in partnership with the range of stakeholders in the problem.

Research and evaluation methods are similar within social-behavioural and social-ecological approaches. However, social ecology, with its reliance on systems theory, adds another level of complexity to evaluation design by attempting to measure system-wide changes from interventions, in addition to changes in target populations. As a result, the evaluation of ecological strategies may emphasize equally qualitative and quantitative techniques (Goodman and Wandersman, 1994). Evaluations of empowerment interventions have relied heavily on qualitative methods (Eng and Parker, 1994), although some projects have included strong quantitative components (Israel *et al.*, 1994). Moreover, empowerment strategies frequently emphasize the involvement of participants in the process of evaluating success of interventions or generation of new findings (often called participatory action research) (Israel *et al.*, 1995).

The three approaches differ most in how they define the outcomes anticipated and deemed acceptable and the audience for research findings. Findings from social-behavioural and social-ecological research are often viewed as providing the basis for needed policy or programmatic change and policy-makers are a primary target audience for results. Empowerment advocates, on the other hand, with their emphasis on involvement of participants in the evaluation process and participatory action research, deem members of the group or community involved as the primary audience for research findings. These categories of approach do not necessarily capture all the nuances in conceptualizing and conducting health promotion research. Nonetheless, they distinguish some fundamental differences in the way investigators in the US are designing and testing interventions thought to be promising for enhancing the public's health.

SUMMARY AND CONCLUSIONS

While the United States has conducted significant research on health promotion and disease prevention, the proportional expenditure on health promotion interventions, compared to medical care, is relatively small with prevention efforts consuming approximately 1 per cent of health-related dollars (Lee and Paxman, 1997). Moreover, much of the research and evaluation effort in health promotion and disease prevention has been based on social and behavioural approaches with emphasis on behaviour and health status outcomes in given populations. Despite its limitations, the social-behavioural approach has contributed substantially to our knowledge of effective settings, strategies, theories and principles, and evaluation methods for health promotion (Clark and McLeroy, 1995).

Major changes occurring in public health and medical care in the United States, including the ageing of the population, rise in health care costs, quest for evidence of effectiveness, evolution of managed care, concern about the quality of care, developments in basic science, consumer trends, and the entry of new players into the prevention arena may serve to strengthen the prevention and health promotion focus in the United States. The relatively recent introduction of alternate frameworks for conceiving of health promotion and implementing interventions, particularly social ecology and empowerment approaches may expand our ideas about prevention to include more emphasis on needed system changes and greater recognition of the effects of social and economic disparities on health.

Notes

1 Sections of this paper are adapted from papers originally appearing in *Health Education Quarterly* 22(3), 1995.
2 The approaches presented in Table 2.1 are for comparison purposes. It is important to recognize that the presentation is illustrative only. There are considerable variations within approaches; for example, social cognitive theory emphasizes a dynamic relationship among self-efficacy, outcome expectation, and social environment variables.

References

Ajzen, I. and Fishbein, M. (1980): *Understanding attitudes and predicting social behavior*. Englewood Cliffs, NJ: Prentice Hall.

Bartholomew, L.K., Parcel, G.S., Seiheimer, D.K., Czyzewski, D., Spinelli, S.H. and Congdon, B. (1991): Development of a health education program to promote the self-management of cystic fibrosis. *Health Education Quarterly* 18: 415–443.

Basch, C.E. (1987): Focus group interview: an under-utilized research technique for improving theory and practice in health education. *Health Education Quarterly*, 14: 411–448.

Becker, M.H. and Maiman, L.A. (1980): Strategies for enhancing patient compliance. *Journal of Community Health* winter (6): 113–135.

Bierer, M.F. and Rigotti, N.A. (1992): Public policy for the control of tobacco-related disease. *Medical Clinics of North America* 76: 515–539.

Borland, R., Owen, N., Hill, D. and Schofield, P. (1991): Predicting attempts and sustained cessation of smoking after the introduction of workplace smoking bans. *Health Psychology* 10(5): 336–342.

Borland, R., Pierce, J.P., Burns, D.M., Gilpin, E., Johnson, M. and Bal, D. (1992): Protection from environmental tobacco smoke in California: the case for a smoke-free workplace. *Journal of the American Medical Association* 268(6): 749–752.

Brownson, R.C., Koffman, D.M., Novotny, T.E., Hughes, R.G. and Eriksen, M.P. (1995): Environmental and policy interventions to control tobacco use and prevent cardiovascular disease. *Health Education Quarterly* 22(4): 478–498.

Burhansstipanov, L. and Dresser, C.M. (1993): *Native American monograph #1: documentation of the cancer research needs of American indians and Alaska natives*. National Cancer Institute. NIH Pub. No. 93–3603.

Christenson, G.M., Gold, R.S., Katz, M. and Kreuter, M.W. (1985): Results of the School Health Education Evaluation. *Journal of School Health* 55(8): 295–355.

Clark, N.M., Evans, D., Zimmerman, B.J., Levison, M.J. and Mellins, R.B. (1994a): Patient and family management of asthma: theory based techniques for the clinician. *Journal of Asthma* 3(16): 427–435.

Clark, N.M., Feldman, C.H., Evans, D., Levison, M.J., Wasilewski, Y. and Mellins, R.B. (1986): The impact of health education on frequency and cost of health care used by low income children with asthma. *Journal of Allergy and Clinical Immunology* 78: 108–115.

Clark, N.M., Janz, N.K., Becker, M.H., Schork, M.A., Wheeler, J., Liang, J., Dodge, J.A., Keteyian, S., Rhoads, K.L. and Santinga, J.T. (1992): Impact of self-management education on the functional health status of older adults with heart disease. *The Gerontologist* 32: 438–443.

Clark, N.M., Janz, N.K., Dodge, J.A. and Garrity, C.R. (1994b): Managing heart disease: a study of the experience of older women. *Journal of the American Medical Women's Association* 49: 202–206.

Clark, N.M., Levison, M.J., Evans, D., Wasilewski, Y., Feldman, C.H. and Mellins, R.B. (1990): Communication within low income families and the management of asthma. *Patient Education and Counselling* 15: 191–210.

Clark, N. and McLeroy, K. (1995): Creating capacity through health education: what we know and what we don't. *Health Education Quarterly* 22(3): 273–289.

Clark, N. and Zimmerman, B.J. (1990): A social cognitive view of self-regulated learning about health. *Health Education and Research* 5(3): 371–379.

Cohen, R.A., VanNostrand, J.F. and Furner, S.E. (eds) (1993): *Chartbook on health data on older Americans: United States, 1992.* National Center for Health Statistics. Vital Health Statistics 3(29).

COMMIT Research Group: Community intervention trial for smoking cessation (COMMIT) (1991): Summary of design and intervention. *Journal of the National Cancer Institute,* 83: 1,620–1,628.

Connell, C.M., Fisher, E.B. Jr and Houston, C.A. (1992): Relationship among social support, diabetes outcomes, and morale for older men and women. *Journal of Ageing and Health* 4: 77–100.

Cook, T.D. and Campbell, D.T. (1979): *Quasi-experimentation: design and Analysis for field settings.* Boston: Houghton Mifflin Co.

Cummings, K.M., Pechacek, T. and Shopland, D. (1994): The illegal sale of cigarettes to U.S. minors: estimates by state. *American Journal of Public Health* 84: 300–302.

Daltroy, L.H., Morlino, C.I. and Liang, M.H. (1989): Preoperative education for total hip and knee replacement patients. *Arthritis Care & Research* 2: S8–15.

Department of Labor (1980): *Protecting people at work: a reader in occupational safety and health.* Washington, DC: United States Government Printing Office.

DiFranza, J.R., Carlson, R.R. and Caisse, R.E. (1992): Reducing youth access to tobacco. *Tobacco Control* 1: 57–58.

DiFranza, J.R., Norwood, B.D., Garnder, D.W. and Tye, J.B. (1987): Legislative efforts to protect children from tobacco. *Journal of the American Medical Association* 257: 3,387–3,389.

Dignan, M., Michielutte, R., Sharp, P., Young, L. and Daniels, L. (1991): Use of process evaluation to guide Forsyth County's project to prevent cervical cancer. *Public Health Reports* 106: 73–77.

Eng, E. (1993): The Save Our Sisters Program: a social network strategy for reaching rural black women. *Cancer* 72(3): 1,071–1,077.

Eng, E. and Parker, E. (1994): Measuring community competence in the Mississippi delta: the interface between program evaluation and empowerment. *Health Education Quarterly* 21(2): 199–220.

Eng, E. and Young, R. (1992): Lay health advisors as community change agents. *Family & Community Health* 15: 24–40.

Evans, D., Clark, N.M. and Feldman, C.H. (1987): School health education programs for asthma. *Clinical Review of Allergy* 5: 207–212.

Farquhar, J.W., Maccoby, N., Wood, P., Alexander, J.K., Breitrose, H., Brown, R.W., Haskell,

W.L., McAlister, A.L., Meyer, A.J., Nash, J.D. and Stern, M.P. (1977): Community education for cardiovascular health. *Lancet* 1: 1,192–1,195.

Fetterman, D.M., Kaftarian, S.J. and Wandersman, A. (1996): *Empowerment evaluation: knowledge and tools for self-assessment and accountability*. Thousand Oaks, CA: Sage Publishing.

Flynn, B.C. (1992): Healthy sites: a model of community change. *Family and Community Health* 15: 13–23.

Forster, J.L., Hourigan, M.E. and Kelder, S. (1992): Locking devices on cigarette vending machines: Evaluation of a city ordinance. *American Journal of Public Health* 82(9): 1,217–1, 219.

Freire, P. (1973): *Education for critical consciousness*. New York: Seabury Press.

Freudenberg, N., (1984): *Not in our backyards! Community action for health and the environment*. New York: Monthly Review Press.

Freudenberg, N., Eng, E., Flay, B., Parcel, G., Rogers, T. and Wallerstein, N. (1995): Strengthening individual and community capacity to prevent disease and promote health: in search of relevant theories and principles. *Health Education Quarterly* 22(3): 290–306.

Freudenberg, N. and Zimmerman, M. (1995): The lessons of AIDS prevention for public health practice, in N. Freudenberg and M. Zimmerman (eds): *AIDS prevention in the community: lessons from the first decade*. Washington, DC: American Public Health Association, 183–197.

German, P.S. and Fried, L.P. (1989): Prevention and the elderly: public health issues and strategies. *Annual Review of Public Health*. Palo Alto, CA: Annual Reviews, Inc., 10: 319–332.

Gielen, A.C., Faden, R.R., O'Campo, P., Kass, N. and Anderson, J. (1994): Women's protective sexual behaviors: a test of the Health Belief Model. *AIDS Education and Prevention* 6(1): 1–11.

Glasgow, R.E., McCaul, K.D. and Fisher, K.J. (1993): Participation in worksite health promotion: A critique of the literature and recommendations for future practice. *Health Education Quarterly* 20: 391–408.

Goodman, R.M. and Wandersman, A. (1994): Forecast: a formative approach to evaluating community coalitions and community-based interventions. *Journal of Community Psychology* CSAP, Special Issue.

Gottlieb, B.H. (1985): Social networks and social support: an overview of research practice, and policy implications. *Health Education Quarterly* 12: 5–22.

Gottlieb, N.H., Lovato, C.Y., Weinstein, R., Green, L.W. and Eriksen, M.P. (1992): The implementation of a restrictive worksite smoking policy in a large decentralized organization. *Health Education Quarterly* 19: 77–100.

Gottlieb, N.H., Wright, D. and Sneden, G.G. (1994): Using PRECEDE/PROCEED for implementation planning: infusion of the Texas 'Top Priority' worksite health promotion program. University of Texas at Austin, unpublished manuscript.

Green, L.W. and Kreuter, M.W. (1991): *Health promotion planning: a diagnostic approach*. Mountain View, CA: Mayfield Publishing Company.

Guttman, N. (1997): Values and ethical dilemmas in public health, communication interventions: An analytic approach. Unpublished manuscript.

Hancock, T. (1993): Health, human development and the community ecosystem: three ecological models. *Health Promotion International* 8: 41–47.

Hanson, W.B. and Graham, J.W. (1991): Preventing alcohol, marijuana, and cigarette use among adolescents: peer pressure resistance training versus establishing conservative norms. *Preventive Medicine* 20: 414–430.

Healthy People: Surgeon General's Report on Health Promotion and Disease Prevention (1979): Washington, DC: US Public Health Service, US Dept of Health, Education, and Welfare, DHEW-PHS-79-55071.

Hollis, J.F., Lichtenstein, E., Vogt, T.M., Stevens, V.J. and Biglan, A. (1993): Nurse assisted counselling for smokers in primary care. *Annals of Internal Medicine* 118(7): 521–525.

Institute of Medicine (1988): *The Future of Public Health*. Washington, DC: National Academy Press.

Inui, T.S., Yourtee, E.L. and Williamson, J.W. (1976): Improved outcomes in hypertension after physician tutorials. *Annals of Internal Medicine* 84: 646–651.

Israel, B.A., Checkoway, B., Schulz, A. and Zimmerman, M.A. (1994): Health education and community empowerment: conceptualizing and measuring perceptions of individual, organizational, and community control. *Health Education Quarterly* 21: 149–170.

Israel, B.A., Cummings, K.M., Dignan, M.B., Heaney, C.A., Perales, D.P., Simons-Morton, B.G. and Zimmerman, M. (1995): Evaluation of health education programs: current assessment and future directions. *Health Education Quarterly* 22(3): 365–389.

Israel, B.A. and Schuman, S.J. (1990): Social support, control and the stress process, in K. Glanz, F.M. Lewis and B.K. Rimer (eds.): *Health behavior and health education*. San Francisco, CA: Jossey-Bass.

Janz, N.K. and Becker, M.H. (1984): The health belief model: a decade later. *Health Education Quarterly* 11: 1–47.

Janz, N.K., Becker, M.H. and Hartman, P.E. (1984): Contingency contracting to enhance patient compliance: a review. *Patient Education and Counselling* 5(4): 165–178.

Jason, L.A., Ji, P.Y., Anes, M.D. and Birkhead, S.H. (1991): Active enforcement of cigarette control laws in the prevention of cigarette sales to minors. *Journal of the American Medical Association* 266: 3,159–3,161.

Jones, L.C. (1986): A meta-analytic study of the effects of childbirth education on the parent–infant relationship. *Health Care for Women International* 7: 357–370.

Kirby, D,, Short, L., Collins, J., Rugg, D., Kolbe, L., Howard, M., Miller, B., Sonenstein, F. and Zabin, L.S. (1994): School-based programs to reduce sexual risk behaviors: a review of effectiveness. *Public Health Reports* 109(3): 339–360.

Kovar, P.A., Allegrante, J.P., MacKenzie, C.R., Peterson, M.G.E., Gutin, B. and Charlson, M.E. (1992): Supervised fitness walking in patients with osteoarthritis of the knee: a randomized, controlled trial. *Annals of Internal Medicine* 116: 529–534.

Lee, P., Benjamin, A.E. and Weber, M.A. (1996): Policies and strategies for health in the United States, in W. Holland, R. Detels and G. Knox (eds): *Oxford Textbook of Public Health*. Oxford: Oxford University Press, 3rd edition.

Lee, P. and Paxman, D. (1997): Reinventing public health. *Annual Review of Public Health* 18: 1–35.

Lewis, F.M. and Daltroy, L.H. (1990): How causal explanations influence health behavior: attribution theory, in K. Glanz, F.M. Lewis and B.K. Rimer (eds): *Health Behavior and Health Education: Theory, Research and Practice*. San Francisco, CA: Jossey-Bass, 92–114.

Lorig, K. and Gonzalez, V. (1992): The integration of theory with practice: a 12-year case study. *Health Education Quarterly* 19: 355–368.

Lorig, K., Konkol, L. and Gonzales, V. (1987): Arthritis patient education: a review of the literature. *Patient Education and Counselling* 10: 207–252.

Lorig, K., Lubeck, D., Kraines, R.G., Seleznick, M. and Holman, H.R. (1985): Outcomes of self-help education for patients with arthritis. *Arthritis & Rheumatism* 28: 680–685.

Luepker, R.V., Murray, D.M., Jacobs, D.R., Mittelmark, M.B., Bracht, N., Carlaw, R., Crow, R., Elmer, P., Finnegan, J., Folsom, A.R., Grimm, R., Hannan, P.J., Jeffrey, R., Lando, H., McGovern, P., Mullis, R., Perry, C.L., Pechacek, T., Pirie, P., Sprafka, J.M., Weisbrod, R. and Blackburn, H. (1994): Community education for cardiovascular disease prevention: risk factor changes in the Minnesota heart health program. *American Journal of Public Health* 84(9): 1,383–1,393.

Marin, G., Burhansstipanov, L., Connell, C.M., Gielen, A.C., Helitzer-Allen, D., Lorig, K., Morisky, D.E., Tenney, M. and Thomas, S. (1995): A research agenda for health education among under-served populations. *Health Education Quarterly* 22(3): 346–364.

Marin, G., Posner, S.F. and Kinyon, J.B. (1993): Alcohol expectancies among Hispanics and non-Hispanic Whites: roles of drinking status and acculturation. *Hispanic Journal of Behavorial Science*, 15: 373–381.

Marin, G., VanOss Marin, B., Otero-Sabogal, R., Sabogal, F. and Perez-Stable, E.J. (1989): The role of acculturation on the attitude, norms and expectations of Hispanic Smokers. *Journal of Cross-Cultural Psychology* 20: 399–415.

McGinnis, J.M. and Foege, W.H. (1993): Actual causes of death in the United States. *JAMA* 270: 2,207–2,212.

McLeroy, K.R., Bibeau, D., Steckler, A. and Glanz, K. (1988): An ecological perspective on health promotion programs. *Health Education Quarterly* 15: 351–377.

McLeroy, K., Clark, N.M., Simons-Morton, B.G., Forster, J., Connell, C.M., Altman, D. and Zimmerman, M. (1995): Creating capacity: establishing a health education research agenda for special populations. *Health Education Quarterly* 22(3): 390–405.

McLeroy, K., Steckler, A., Kegler, M., Burdine, J. and Wizotsky, M. (1994): Community coalitions for health promotion: summary and further reflections. *Health Education Research: Theory and Practice* 9(1): 1–11.

Mechanic, D. (1989): Socio-economic status and health: the problem, in J.P. Bunker, D.S. Gomby and B.H. Kehrer (eds): *Pathways to health: the role of social factors*. Menlo Park, CA: Henry J. Kaiser Family Foundation.

Michielutte, R., Dignan, M.B., Wells, H.B., Young, L.D., Jackson, D.S. and Sharp, P.C. (1989): Development of a community cancer education program: the Forsyth County, NC, cervical cancer prevention project. *Public Health Reports* 104: 542–551.

Mittlemark, M.B., Hunt, M.K., Heath, G.W. and Schmid, T.L. (1993): Realistic outcomes: lessons from community-based research and demonstration programs for the prevention of cardiovascular diseases. *Journal of Public Health Policy* 14: 437–462.

Montgomery, K. (1993): The Harvard Alcohol Project: promoting the designated driver on television, in T.E. Backer, E.M. Rogers *Organizational aspects of health communication campaigns: what works*. Newbury Park, CA: Sage Publications.

Morisky, D.E., Malotte, C.K., Choi, P., Davidson, P., Rigler, S., Sugland, B. and Langer, M. (1990): A patient education program to improve adherence rates with anti-tuberculosis drug regimens. *Health Education Quarterly* 17: 253–267.

Mullen, P.D., Evans, D., Forster, J., Gottlieb, N.H., Kreuter, M., Moon, R., O'Rourke, T. and Strecher, V.J. (1995): Settings as an important dimension in health education/promotion policy, programs, and research. *Health Education Quarterly*, 22(3): 329–345.

Mullen, P.D., Laville, E.A., Biddle, A.K. and Lorig, K. (1987): Efficacy of psycho-educational interventions on pain, depression, and disability with arthritic adults: a meta-analysis. *Journal of Rheumatology* 14 (Suppl. 15): 33–39.

Mullen, P.D., Mains, D.A. and Velez, R. (1992): A meta-analysis of controlled trials of cardiac patient education. *Patient Education and Counselling* 19: 1,443–62.

Mullen, P.D., McCuan, R.A. and Iverson, D.C. (1986): Evaluation of health education and promotion programs: a review of qualitative approaches. *Advances in Health Education Promotion* 1: 467–498.

National Cancer Institute (August, 1993): *The impact of cigarette excise taxes on smoking among children and adults*. Summary Report of a National Cancer Institute Expert Panel. Rockville, MD. Cancer Control Science Program, Division of Cancer Prevention and Control.

National Center for Health Statistics (1990): *Health United States 1989: and prevention profile*. (DHHS Pub. No. PHS 90–1,232).

Overbo, B., Ryan, M., Jackson, K. and Hutchinson, K. (1994): The homeless prenatal program: a model for empowering homeless pregnant women. *Health Education Quarterly* 21: 187–198.

Padgett, D., Mumford, E., Hynes, M. and Carter, R. (1988): Meta-analysis of the effects of educational and psychosocial interventions on management of diabetes mellitus. *Journal of Clinical Epidemiology* 41(10): 1,007–1,030.

Parcel, G.S., Perry, C.L. and Taylor, W.C. (1990): Beyond demonstration: diffusion of health promotion innovations, in N. Bracht (ed.): *Health promotion at the community level.* Newbury Park, CA: Sage, 229–252.

Pelletier, K.R. (1993): A review and analysis of the health and cost-effective outcome studies of comprehensive health promotion and disease prevention programs at the worksite. *American Journal of Health Promotion* 50–62.

Perez-Stable, E.J., VanOss Marin, B. and Marin, G. (1993): A comprehensive smoking cessation program for the San Francisco Bay Area Latino community: Programa Latino Para Dejar de Fumar. *American Journal of Health Promotion* 7(6): 430–442, 475.

Pierce, J.P., Evans, N., Farkas, A., Cavin, S.W. and Berry, C. (1994): *Tobacco use in California: an evaluation of the tobacco control program 1989–1993.* La Jolla, CA: University of California, San Diego.

Pierce, J.P., Mills, S.L., Shopland, D.R. *et al.* (1992): Accessibility of cigarettes to youths aged 12–17 years – United States, 1989. *Morbidity and Mortality Weekly Report* 41: 485–488.

Prochaska, J.O. and DiClemente, C.C. (1986): Towards a comprehensive model of change, in W.R. Miller and N. Heather (eds): *Treating addictive behavior.* New York: Plenum, 3–27.

Rice, R.E. and Atkin, C.K. (eds.) (1990): *Public communication campaigns* (2nd edition). Newbury Park, CA: Sage Publications.

Rigotti, N.A., Stoto, M.A. and Schelling, T.C. (1994): Do businesses comply with a no-smoking law? Assessing the self-enforcement approach. *Preventive Medicine* 23: 223–229.

Rivo, M., Gray, K., Whitaker, M., Coward, R., Biburd, L., Timoll, M., Curry, C. and Tuckson, R. (1992): Implementing PATCH in public housing communities: the District of Columbia experience. *Journal of Health Education* 23: 148–152.

Rogers, E. (1993): *Diffusion of innovations.* New York: The Free Press.

Rosenstock, I.M., Stergachis, A. and Heaney, C. (1986): Evaluation of smoking prohibition policy in a health maintenance organization. *American Journal of Public Health* 76(8): 1,014–1,015.

Ross, J., Nelson, G. and Kolbe, L. (1991): Teenage health teaching modules evaluation. *Journal of School Health* 61(1): 19–42.

Rosser, S.V. (1991): Perspectives: AIDS and women. *AIDS Education Prevention,* 3(3): 230–240.

Simons-Morton, D.C., Simons-Morton, B.G., Parcel, G.S. and Bunker, J.F. (1988): Influencing personal and environmental conditions for community health: a multi-level intervention model. *Family and Community Health* August: 25–35.

Skinner, C.S., Strecher, V.J. and Hosper, H. (1993): Physician recommendations for mammography: do tailored messages make a difference? *American Journal of Public Health* 84(1): 43–49.

Sorensen, G., Glasgow, R.E. and Corbett, K. (1992): Compliance with worksite non-smoking policies: baseline results from the COMMIT study of worksites. *American Journal of Health Promotion* 7(2): 103–109.

Special Issue (Summer, 1994a): Community empowerment, participatory education, and health – Part I. *Health Education Quarterly* 21(2).

Special Issue (Fall, 1994b): Community empowerment, participatory education, and health – Part II. *Health Education Quarterly* 21(3).

Steckler, A. (1989): The use of qualitative evaluation methods to test internal validity. *Evaluation and the Health Professions* 12: 115–133.

Steckler, A., Allegrante, J.P., Altman, D., Brown, R., Burdine, J.N., Goodman, R.M. and Jorgensen, C. (1995): Health education intervention strategies: recommendations for future research. *Health Education Quarterly,* 22(3): 307–328.

Stewart, M.J. (1989): Social support: diverse theoretical perspectives. *Social Science and Medicine* 28(12): 275–282.

Stillman, F.A., Bone, L.R., Rand, C., Levine, D.M. and Becker, D.M. (1993): Heart, body, and soul: a church-based smoking-cessation program for urban African Americans. *Preventive Medicine* 22(3): 335–349.

Stokols, D. (1996): Translating social ecological theory into guidelines for community health promotion. *American Journal of Health Promotion* 10(4): 282–298.

Stokols, D. (1992): Establishing and maintaining health environments: towards a social ecology of health promotion. *American Psychology* 47: 6–22.

Stone, E.J., McGraw, S.A. and Osgannian, S.K. (1994): Process evaluation in the multicenter child and adolescent trial for cardiovascular health (CATCH). *Health Education Quarterly* (S2) S1–148.

Strecher, V.J. (1982): Improving physician–patient interactions: A review. *Patient Counselling and Health Education*, 4: 129–136.

Strecher, V.J., Kreuter, M.W., Den Boer, D.J., Kobrins, Hospers, H.J. and Skinner, C.S. (1994): The effects of computer-tailored smoking cessation messages in family practice settings. *Journal of Family Practice* 39(3): 262–270.

Uba, L. (1992): Cultural barriers to health care for Southeast Asian refugees. *Public Health Reports* 107: 544–548.

US Department of Health and Human Services (1992): *Smoking and health in the Americas*. Atlanta, GA, US Department of Health and Human Services, Centers for Disease Control and Prevention (DHHS Pub. No. CDC 92–8419).

US Department of Health and Human Services (1994): *Reducing tobacco use among young people: a report of the Surgeon General*. Atlanta, GA, Public Health Service, Centers for Disease Control and Prevention, National Center for Chronic Disease Prevention and Health Promotion, Office on Smoking and Health.

US Surgeon General (1979): *Report on health promotion and disease prevention*. HRP-0030741/3, p. 264.

US Surgeon General (1989): *Reducing the health consequences of smoking: 25 years of progress*. Report of the Surgeon General. Washington, DC: U. S. Department of Health and Human Services, Public Health Service, Centers for Disease Control, Center for Chronic Disease Prevention and Health Promotion, Office on Smoking and Health. (DHHS Pub. No. CDC 89–8411).

Wallack, L. (1990): Mass communication and health promotion, in R.E. Rice and C.E. Atkin (eds): *Public communication campaigns* (2nd edition). Newbury Park, CA: Sage Publications.

Wallerstein, N. and Bernstein, E. (1988): Empowerment education: Freire's ideas adapted to health education. *Health Education Quarterly* 15: 379–394.

Wallerstein, N. and Bernstein, E. (1994): Introduction to community empowerment, participatory education, and health. *Health Education Quarterly* 21(2): 141–148.

Wallston, K.A. and Wallston, B.S. (1978): Locus of control and health. *Health Education Monographs* 6: 107–117.

Walter, H. and Wynder, E. (1989): The development, implementation, evaluation, and future directions of chronic disease prevention programs for children: the 'Know Your Body' studies. *Preventive Medicine* 8(1): 59–71.

Wang, C. and Burris, M.A. (1994): Empowerment through photo novella: portraits of participation. *Health Education Quarterly* 21: 171–186.

Warner, K.E. (1986): Smoking and health implications of a change in the federal cigarette excise tax. *Journal of the American Medical Association* 255: 1,028–1,032.

Watkins, E.L., Harlan, C., Eng, E., Gansky, S.A., Gehan, D. and Larson, K. (1994): Assessing the effectiveness of lay health advisors with migrant farm workers. *Family & Community Health* 16: 72–87.

Whelton, P.K., Perneger, T.V., Klag, M.J. and Brancati, F.L. (1992): Epidemiology and prevention of blood pressure-related renal disease. *Journal of Hypertension* 10 (Suppl. 7) S77–S84.

Wigal, J.K., Creer, T.L. *et al.* (1990): A critique of 19 self-management programs of childhood asthma: part II, development and evaluation of the programs. *Pediatr. Asthma, Allergy, and Immunology* 4: 17–39.

Winett, R., King, A.C. and Altman, D.G. (1989): *Health psychology and public health: an integrative perspective*. New York: Pergamon Press.

Chapter 3

Evaluating health promotion in four key settings

Cecily Kelleher

DEFINITIONS AND CONTEXT

Much has been written about the rationale for health promotion, including discussion about what specific strategies should be promoted, in what context, for whom intervention is appropriate and how it might be undertaken most effectively. The Ottawa Charter (WHO, 1986) has been widely adopted as the framework for modern health promotion, and its core definition is primarily one of enablement. The Charter emphasised the five different means of promoting health, through healthy public policy, community participation, personal skills development, re-oriented heath services and by means of the creation of supportive environments. Perhaps a critical factor about Ottawa was that it succeeded in moving thinking on from the prevalent paradigm of individual risk factor intervention to promote health. It follows, therefore, that a quality health promotion intervention should be measured now by whether or not it had measurably enabled individuals or communities to take control of their own health (Ziglio, 1997). This, however, is rarely the parameter by which health promotion interventions are judged. In very recent years serious consideration has been given to the issue of quality in health promotion and a working group established to set out standards for quality (Deccache, 1997; MacDonald, 1997; Rootman, 1997; Saan, 1997; Ovretveit, 1996). This chapter will concern itself with this issue as it applies to settings-based initiatives, particularly in an Irish context.

Since the original meeting in Ottawa, there have been three further major WHO sponsored conferences: on healthy public policy in Adelaide (WHO, 1988), in Sundsvall (WHO, 1991), where the so called settings approach was first crystallised and in Jakarta. The declaration from the Sundsvall meeting emphasised the appropriateness of creating supportive environments to enable individuals to take control of their health; indeed throughout the 1980s the World Health Organization-sponsored Healthy Cities initiative was established successfully across the globe. Key micro settings included school, workplace, hospitals and primary care. Since then this concept has been considerably expanded to include a range of other environments or settings, including islands

(Nutbeam, 1996) and prisons (Squires and Strobl, 1997). More recent World Health Organisation initiatives include the Mega country strategy. In Jakarta in July of 1997 at a meeting entitled 'New Players for a New Era', the socio-political basis of health promotion was further expanded to embrace the many partners and agencies whose co-operation will be required to promote health and well-being at a global level, including the private as well as the statutory and Non Governmental Organisation (NGO) sector and most potent of all, the media. As the parameters for health promotion have expanded so too have the challenges to implement and evaluate such initiatives (Davies, 1996; Tones, 1997) and to define the principles on which such developments are justified (Dean, 1996; Kelleher, 1995; McLeroy et al., 1993; McQueen, 1996).

While health promotion originally had its theoretical base in the work undertaken by the parent disciplines associated with it, including epidemiology, psychology, sociology, anthropology, social marketing and communications, increasingly there has been a search for grounded theories of health promotion itself. This multi-disciplinary Tower of Babel would have a challenge in any context but in the matter of human health and its determinants those challenges are immense (Kelleher, 1996). It is likely that there is no one right answer and no single means of achieving population health, which has contributed to the debate and confusion around this issue, particularly by those who have not adopted the thinking behind the Ottawa framework. Increasingly, the literature has focused on the paradigms which inform health promotion. This debate was originally seen to be almost dichotomous. The reductionist or mechanistic approach to health and illness, exemplified by epidemiology, seeks to quantify precisely the often inter-related risk factors at an individual level across populations; this method has informed many of the means of evaluating community health promotion initiatives to date, particularly in the case of disease specific interventions. The complex inter-relationship of the many factors that influence health has been difficult to define but, increasingly, the more sophisticated investigators in the reductionist school have proposed factors along the life-course that inter-relate with each other, but can indeed be quantified. An example is the debate about early life influences on coronary heart disease (Barker and Osmond, 1986; Davey-Smith et al., 1997).

More recently, the social science position has reasserted itself and the resultant literature has focused on the holistic nature of health and well-being and the need to examine issues from a constructivist paradigm (Antonovsky, 1993; Antonovsky, 1996; Labonte, 1989; Nutbeam, 1997). This literature is much more sociological in orientation and seeks to refine what we have in common as societies that could be capitalised upon to create a social fabric conducive to health. Measures of success in this context integrate and learn from the process of promoting health as much as the outcome. A core problem is that even those who accept a widely-based socio-political explanation of ill health are reluctant to assert that there is any determinant of good health per se. Writers such as Ilona Kickbusch (Kickbusch, 1996; 1997) have supported consistently the notion that health promoting situations can be created as part of the fabric of everyday life, which is essentially a political statement for the organisation of our societies. However, what do we know about positive influences on health at a social or individual level? The concept of Salutogenesis was first enunciated by Antonovsky (Antonovsky, 1993; Antonovsky, 1996). This proposes that we have measured health largely by its absence to date, and that there may well be positive factors that protect individuals, even in the face of adverse circumstances. This he attempted to quantify as a sense of social coherence and evolved a measurable scale that he applied in different contexts. Criticism levelled at salutogenesis includes the notion that it is over simplistic given the wide range of disease processes (Siegrist, 1993; Davey-Smith and Egger, 1996 and 1997) and variety of inter-related risk factors and that the scale itself does not appreciably differ from a range of similar socio-psychological constructs. However even in epidemiological terms, all things being equal, some do and some do not succumb to specific illnesses and it is within such groups with closely similar conventional risk factor profiles that we should be studying this issue. It may be a matter of probability who succumbs or who doesn't, or it may be to do with as yet unquantifiable elements more familiarly explored in the humanities and literature generally, such as spirituality, love and hope. This is not traditional epidemiological territory but it has not been well explored in the health promotion literature either, though there are signs of increasing interest (Bobak and Marmot, 1995; Bunker et al., 1996; Bygren et al., 1996; Hawks et al., 1995).

Traditionally health service evaluation derives from the clinical experimental model of investigation and involves the setting of pre-formulated or a priori goals or timeframe, the establishment of a control, comparison or reference situation, measurement by intention to participate and ideally the use of random allocation to the intervention. The proponents of evidence-based medicine accept this approach as a kind of gold standard. A sometimes complementary but essentially alternative approach is a formative evaluation, which is often more realistic in field research. This includes the need to assimilate feedback based on the impact of the intervention in order to improve it, to be prepared for agenda setting by participants themselves rather than the research team and the concentration on quality and process of delivery. The potential contradiction has led to considerable confusion in the literature about what can be called models of good practice (Nutbeam et al., 1990). The situation has also been complicated by the development of disciplinary rivalries. Public health practitioners worldwide are mainly medically qualified, have moved more slowly towards multi-discipline work and have for the most part in most countries a clear role of health protection and disease prevention within a structured health-service setting. Informing theory is mainly based on an epidemiological model with some public policy or advocacy components. Its dominant methodologies are quantitative. Health promotion practice on the other hand has grown since the 1980s from the health education tradition, has been multi-disciplinary from the outset and involves a range of disparate practitioners from all kinds of settings. It has lacked a natural means of operation because of its ambitious multi-sectoral nature and hence tended for practical purposes to become compartmentalised in the general mind as a lifestyle education function. Health promotion has been an applied social science whose theoretical framework has developed from a psychology, anthropology and sociology base. Its emerging methodologies are qualitative or a triangular combination. Up to now, it has been a movement or a synthesis of different disciplinary ideas applied in different contexts, but at this stage there is considerable question as to whether health promotion is a discrete discipline and has specific informing theories of its own; this is why those like salutogenesis have gained increasing importance. To date however, there has been little empirical evidence that such theories inform mass health promotion movements in any practical sense. A review of health behaviour professionals in the United States indicated remarkable consensus for models of intentions to change, self-efficacy and social support (Love *et al.*, 1996) as influences for lifestyle programs but this has potential limitations in the socio-political and indeed ecological paradigm (Green *et al.*, 1996) that Ottawa Charter health promotion entails. It is appropriate to consider the quality of the settings approach to health promotion in the context of this debate.

SETTINGS FOR HEALTH PROMOTIONS

Key features of a settings-based approach include consultation on needs (which should be wide ranging, bottom-up in nature and client led), the formulation of an intervention in the context of the setting, a decision on the timeframe and anticipated outcome, some kind of evaluation which might be either summative or formative or a variant of both, and an aspiration that the project should be integrated into the setting in a fixed time scale in a seamless way. In Ireland, at the Centre for Health Promotion Studies, we have undertaken a number of studies in the three broad areas: schools, workplace and primary care. We have also been involved in various community-based projects. I would like to review some of this evidence in addition to more generally published studies in the literature.

School settings

How well have schools-based interventions been evaluated? Though there is a vast literature on every kind of health education initiative over the years on all sorts of topics (many successfully attaining their objectives), health based interventions have largely borrowed from traditional experimental or epidemiological designs for outcome evaluations. In a nutshell, what health professionals, especially doctors, read about health education is couched in and judged according to this paradigm. This has its disadvantages since the general educational literature itself has a quite different focus and has not adapted to this kind of behavioural quantitative approach in any other subject area. As an example of the constraints placed on health promotion by such an approach, Nutbeam *et al.* (1993) reported on a well designed study of smoking-behaviour follow-up among never smokers according to interventions based on materials derived from the Minnesota and Norwegian experience. They found no difference in current smoking rates compared with controls in either the two intervention groups or a combined intervention group. An examination of the programs however, reveals their modest nature. The Smoking and Me program from the Minnesota smoking prevention program targeted 12–13 year olds, averaged five lessons, included a day-long teacher training and had a focus on social consequences; peer, family or media influences. The Family-Smoking Education project targets 11–12 year olds, averages three hours for delivery, includes a booklet for pupils and leaflet for parents, and has a focus on the immediate health impact of smoking. Is it so surprising (Kelleher and Dineen, 1993) that no effects were seen? The authors themselves were clearly aware of the difficulties inherent in such a study and said so in their conclusions. Smoking is so obviously a multi-faceted behaviour that reliance on school health education alone is over simplistic, particularly where the interventions were minimal and project-oriented. The interaction with socio-economic circumstances was not developed in the study and indeed Nutbeam and Aaro (1991) have also shown that pupils with a negative attitude to school are more likely to smoke and presumably less likely to be receptive to intervention. It should be remembered however that these programs were successful in the context of their original development, though not when exported to a different context, pointing up the need for an appropriate educational environment in which to tackle topic specific programs. Our own evaluation of a life-skills program for health promotion in our North-Western Health Board Region in Ireland, based on a self-empowerment model which has run in second level schools for over 12 years, focused on health behaviours, health indicators, health knowledge and personal characteristics (Nic Gabhainn and Kelleher, 1995). That study showed differing effects on smoking and alcohol behaviours and also clear evidence of interaction with social class and gender.

The European Health-Promoting School program sponsored by the World Health Organisation, Council of Europe and the European Union, focuses on the school as a setting, which therefore includes curriculum development, a strong emphasis on an appropriate school ethos for personal development and liaison between family and community. There has been a clear recognition of the cultural, political and organisational differences in different countries, all of which have to be taken account of in program delivery (Parson *et al.*, 1997). To date, there has been no major outcome evaluation published and several impact evaluations are presently in progress (Nic Gabhainn and Kelleher, 1997;

The Health Promoting School Conference, 1997). Similarly in Australia, results are awaited (Booth and Samdai, 1997). The model will specifically not be based primarily on behavioural outcome measures since it is far closer to a mainstream educational program than previous school health initiatives. While intuitively this would appear to be the appropriate educational approach, we await published evaluations on which to measure the quality of programs, and it is clear that operational criteria for quality will need to be developed and agreed before we can say that the programs are a success and generalise the findings. From what we know of school-based studies, we may infer for the present that the programs must be sustained over the entire curriculum, that the school environment and ethos is crucial, that the fostering of self-efficacy is probably as important as self-esteem and that there are gender differences of which account must be taken. It is quite clear that further evidence needs to be accumulated to confirm these conclusions, particularly since there is little in the way of traditional experimental or quasi-experimental evidence to support the benefit, but we do have process and educational data to support the strategy and should be careful how the position is interpreted.

Workplace settings

Workplace studies have now been ongoing in various countries since the mid-1970s (Anderson and Staufacker, 1996; Eickhoff-Shemek and Ryan, 1995; Goetzel *et al.*, 1996; Heaney and Goetzel, 1997; Shephard, 1996). They are mainly lifestyle oriented, using active (or participative) rather than passive (or social change) approaches. This is notably so in the United States where health maintenance has become increasingly a part of health insurance schemes, and where there is a clear focus on lifestyle intervention. There are held to be four generations of programs at this stage (Wilson *et al.*, 1996a, 1996b): programs offered for reasons unrelated to health, those that focus on single intervention of a particular risk factor or behaviour targeted towards one population, a variety of interventions aimed at a range of risk factors for all employees and a comprehensive approach to the working environment incorporating all activities and policies with a likely impact on health and in liaison with the community. The workplace is a natural setting in which to reach individuals and since health promotion concerns itself with equity the variation in health status seen according to social class and occupation is important (Chu *et al.*, 1997). However little has, to date, been published on major settings-based evaluations using more broad ranging health promotion criteria, and few have focused in any serious way on working conditions as an indirect effector of lifestyle behaviour decisions. Such fourth generation studies, in line with health promotion principles will need to be undertaken. Over the last year the *American Journal of Health Promotion* has undertaken a systematic review of effectiveness of existing programs using a rating system that prioritises the randomised controlled trial and that evaluates both individual studies and categories of studies as weak, suggestive, indicative, acceptable or conclusive (Wilson *et al.*, 1996a, 1996b). The results are more positive than might be realised (O'Donnell, 1996). Pelletier (1996) believes that such initiatives can be cost effective, if comprehensively delivered. At a topic specific level there is some variation (Eddy *et al.*, 1997; Eickhoff-Shemek and Ryan, 1995; Glanz *et al.*, 1996; Heaney and Goetzel, 1997; Hennrikus and Jeffery, 1997; Murphy, 1996; Roman and Blum, 1996). Hypertension control programs, for instance, are conclusively effective, weight control programs are indicative but nutrition/cholesterol programs are suggestive rather than clearly indicative. Fielding (1996), in a commentary, identifies the areas for development which include a more concerted focus on organisational issues, a move to involve differing kinds of work environments and the need for operational guidelines.

Again, as in the school setting, it is clear that workplace based studies, which focus on lifestyle interventions on their own, may not always be effective. Perhaps the largest scale and best designed smoking intervention program is that of the COMMIT study (1995). For resource reasons it is unlikely that anything similar will ever be replicated elsewhere (Susser, 1995). This program, however, focused particularly on one lifestyle risk factor, and while it was multi-sectoral in impact utilising public education, organised community events, worksites and education resources, nonetheless, it was mainly a personal skills based initiative. The overall results were disappointing, but with some desired effects in some subgroups. There was for instance a small but significant effect on smoking cessation rate in light to moderate smokers. Are we still treating the problem of smoking in social terms the way we did in the early 1960s and 1970s? There are three issues in smoking: how to deter young and/or poor people from starting in a way that takes account of their reasons and circumstances, particularly women (Graham and Hunt, 1994; Kelleher, 1991; O'Connor *et al.*, 1997); how to influence smokers who are not physically dependent but who choose to smoke as a social statement; and how to help heavy smokers, particularly those with health problems. It is likely at this stage that the proportion of smokers still remaining in the population will not respond to traditional means of smoking cessation support, developed when the prevalence of smoking was higher, and using participation methods suited best to those in general control of their lives, particularly middle-class people; those taking it up now may be doing do for different reasons (Graham and Hunt, 1994; Lynch, 1995, O'Connor *et al.*, 1997). Smoking is a social signal and a barometer of empowerment as well as a health hazard and our response to the issue in the next century will test the subtlety of emerging health promotion initiatives.

We undertook a three-year lifestyle intervention program in the workplace which involved a survey, a one-year intervention and the follow-up evaluation. This was undertaken in industry, the health sector and in a large academic institution including both students and academics (Fleming *et al.*, 1997; Hope *et al.*, 1997; Hope and Kelleher, 1995). The program had a particular focus for blue collar women. At baseline, we found clear class related differences in a range of lifestyle behaviours, which were not unexpected. We specifically focused on organisational issues and services as part of the needs assessment with a view to planning programs according to expressed preferences of employees. For instance, there were a number of dietary patterns of interest (Fleming *et al.*, 1997); those who were regular fish eaters were far more likely to belong to the affluent social classes. Women and men reported different obstacles to dietary change, many practical in nature. Younger women were the only group who were not particularly pressurised by the preferences of other family measures in relation to their dietary behaviours. In our case, we opted for a varying intervention program across cancer-linked risk factors in each of the settings. In the case of nurses for instance (Hope *et al.*, 1997), passive strategies such as improved canteen facilities or no smoking policies were more feasible and better received and the nurses themselves favoured mental health initiatives. In the workplace lifestyle may be a signal as well as a cause of ill health and the solution lies beyond the scope of a three year demonstration project. It can however contribute to the impetus for change. A source of considerable stress for student nurses was second year when they moved into hospitals, which correlated with adverse behaviour change. Since then we have completely re-structured nurse education programs in Ireland and it will be interesting to see what effect this has in subsequent study.

Health needs of blue and white collar workers and of women and men are different and indeed studies consistently show that patterns of ill health are more prevalent among workers in low control jobs (Bosma *et al.*, 1997), but yet there remains a perception that programs should deal with 'executive stress' and a strong focus on individual participation. Social support may not be enough (Terborg *et al.*, 1995) if it does not extend to needed organisational change. Interventions in the workplace are particularly problematic in any case, in that it is difficult to achieve any kind of experimental study design for feasibility reasons. The traditional adversarial labour relations situation of worker and manager leads to challenges in communication, networking and decision-making. This may explain in part why even in affluent countries like North America where employers have a vested interest in worker health it has often proved difficult to mount classical epidemiological studies. Despite the fact that the process of change in the workplace may be crucial in the degree of co-operation, compliance and likely effectiveness of the program, published reports focus almost exclusively on outcome or impact factors. Systematic review shows very different results in different countries and organisations, which may well be dependent on the success of implementing the intervention. To make progress in the workplace, the holistic approach to a health promoting environment may be the best option.

Our best intuitive guess at present about the health promoting workplace is that interventions will only be effective if the environment is generally conducive to health and well-being, that so called passive strategies are more feasible than active ones, and that individual behaviour based programs, whether for smoking cessation or stress management, must also take account of the wider environment. The evidence points to facilitation for blue collar workers particularly, who have less discretion and control at work than white collar workers. For example, people in hazardous work are more likely to smoke (Sorensen *et al.*, 1996). There has to be support from management and ownership by participants, and the cultural factors are so diverse, that it would be difficult to operationalise quality-based workplace interventions. There remains much to be done in this area, particularly in smaller-scale enterprises, or in non-industrial workplaces, which are the main employment settings worldwide, but we should not dismiss the positive evidence accumulated thus far.

Primary care settings

The scope for primary care is enormous but more heterogeneous than any other area so it is appropriate to focus on a particular organisational setting, on general practice based studies, which are relevant to the United Kingdom and Ireland. In these islands, a vocationally trained family doctor sets up a general service, often with partners and with other health professional support and back-up. Traditionally, there is no direct access to specialist hospital services except in an acute emergency. This has led to the conclusion that since most of the population avail of such services, and do so for a range of health care, it should form a focus point for more proactive health mainte-nance services. A large number of short-term intervention studies have been undertaken in the United Kingdom (UK), particularly since so called health promotion initiatives became part of the contractual relationship between GPs and government. The Family Heart Study (1994) for instance, which involved a relatively intensive nurse counselling intervention program, reported among participants a 4 per cent decrease in reported smoking, modest reduc-tion of 1 kg in weight, a small reduction in systolic and diastolic blood pres-sure, a negligible change in total cholesterol, which it was estimated led to an overall cardiovascular disease risk reduction according to the Dundee score of about 12 per cent. The authors concluded that their intervention was more sophisticated than the present contractual arrangements for health promo-tion in general practice in the UK, which therefore meant that the present national strategy could not be justified and that it was important there should be rigorous evaluation of such interventions. They suggested a focus on high risk individuals, since the gain for individuals generally was modest given the intervention resource cost. They also concluded that primary care alone could not provide a population approach to reducing CHD risks, so that more so-phisticated public health policies were needed. A recently published meta-analysis sponsored by the Health Education Authority in the UK (Ebrahim and Davey-Smith, 1997) concluded similarly that lifestyle intervention pro-grams in a primary care setting (which included both general practice and workplace) yielded a small gain at individual level, and hence should be reviewed in favour of wider social change strategies. However, if one looks at the health promotion targets more closely, such conclusions seem very pessimistic in both relative and absolute terms. In an Irish context, for instance, the first health promotion target in our national strategy is to develop more settings based approaches (Table 3.1). The smoking target in Ireland is to reduce the percentage of those who smoke by at least 1 percentage point per year, so that more than 80 per cent of those 15 and over are non-smokers by the year 2000. Repeated studies in primary care have shown that such a target is achievable with relatively modest intervention (Baxter *et al.*, 1997; Russell *et al.*, 1979) and indeed the Family Heart Study is well within such limits. The challenge remains the class differences in smoking and the core issue is whether the diminution of such a gradient will be achieved by social reform alone, by health education in any setting including primary care or by a combination of such approaches. Up to now no one has formulated a scientific study ambitious enough to test such a hypothesis.

A decision is crucially dependent on available infrastructure. In an Irish setting, there are major constraints in any case to health promotion in general practice, in that up to 70 per cent of Irish doctors work single handed with a minimal secretarial backup and no available practice nurse. We presently have an on-going project on health promotion for children which looks at the combined effects of schools and general practice health education (O'Donnell *et al.*, 1997). It is targeted at 8–15 year olds and their families, is a randomised study by practice and factorial in design including either opportunistic or recall programs for family members, delivered by either a doctor or a nurse. The findings are not yet complete, but a preliminary examination of attendance rates in the various practices shows that the more successful groups were nurses' clinics, rather than doctors' clinics, particularly where there was a structured recall invitation. We also found a clear class gradient, like many other studies, in that those in the higher socio-economic groups were more likely to attend. It can be seen that though the effects of general practice based studies are modest, they can contribute to national targets, and that indeed there is consistent evidence from such interventions that concerted preventive medicine programs could have an effective result.

However such programs fall very short of the aspiration for a health promoting health centre (Cainan *et al.*, 1986). Such a centre would be client centred, participative and would act as a focal point in the community for a range of health promoting initiatives across the social and medical spectrum. Health professionals working in such a centre would see advocacy for social change in their area as part of their function. There is therefore a larger question which concerns the attitudes of physicians to health promotion generally and to primary care based health education and preventive medicine in particular. It is quite clear that physicians are influential on public opinion, and their scepticism confuses the general public (Nic Gabhainn and Kelleher, 1996). At present all the debate in the medical literature in these islands equates health promotion

Table 3.1 Health promotion targets in the Republic of Ireland

Area	Targets
General	To develop health promotion programs in school, community, workplace and health service settings so as to promote health at local level
Smoking	To reduce the percentage of those who smoke by at least 1 percentage point per year so that more than 80 per cent of the population aged 15 years and over are non-smokers by the year 2000
Alcohol	To promote moderation in the consumption of alcohol and to reduce the risks to physical, mental and family health that can arise from alcohol misuse To ensure that within the next years, 75 per cent of the population aged 15 years and over knows and understands the recommended sensible limits for alcohol consumption. While these limits are subject to ongoing research, the present international consensus is 14 units per week for a woman and 21 units for a man To reduce substantially over the next 10 years the proportion of those who exceed the recommended sensible limits for alcohol consumption
Nutrition and diet	To educate and motivate Irish people to eat a wide variety of foods in line with current recommendations as illustrated in the Food Pyramid To encourage the achievement and maintenance of a healthy weight through healthy eating and regular exercise To encourage a reduction in total fat intake to no more than 36 per cent of energy (as fat) by the year 2005 and to attain an appropriate balance of fats To achieve a moderate reduction of 10 per cent in the percentage of people who are overweight and a reduction of 10 per cent in the percentage of people who are obese by the year 2005 (this target has been set understanding the difficulties associated with reducing overweight and maintaining a healthy weight)
Exercise	To achieve a 30 per cent increase in the proportion of the population aged 15 and over who engage in an accumulated 30 minutes of light physical exercise most days of the week by the year 2000 To achieve a 20 per cent increase in the proportion of the population age 15 and over who engage in moderate exercise for at least 20 minutes, three times a week by the year 2000
Cholesterol	To achieve a situation where 75 per cent of the population in the 35–64 age group will have a blood pressure of less than 140/10mm Hg by the year 2005 To achieve a reduction in mean serum cholesterol in the 35–65 year age group from a present level of 5.6mmol/L to 5.2mmol/L by the year 2005
Accidents	To achieve a reduction of 10 per cent in mortality due to accidents within the next 10 years and a significant reduction in morbidity particularly among children

Source: Department of Health (1994, 1995).

with biomedical lifestyle initiatives and the results at this level are presented as none too impressive (Ebrahim and Davey-Smith, 1997; Family Heart Study Group, 1994; Nutbeam *et al.*, 1993). Doctors do need to be supportive but may not be the most effective providers of health education and may be prepared to refer for more sophisticated counselling as necessary. They should not be the only channel for lifestyle health promotion. Their potential role is to collaborate with other primary carers, particularly nurses, to advocate health promotion in its real sense at a policy level. There is doubtless an opportunity resources cost to such programs. Many doctors in these islands argue for instance that their present limited activities are at the expense of treatment services and are in any case more appropriate to public health physicians. If so, this is a health services research question worthy of a proper cost effectiveness analysis. On the other hand vocational training for general practitioners may be much more sympathetic to a health promoting service in its truest sense since such training encourages continuity of care over the life course and management of specific illness in a wider context of the patient's circumstances. Indicators of quality service in this respect would be highly valuable and could be developed.

Community settings

Finally, what about community action programs? Again, such programs evolved from a quasi-experimental model, were based around lifestyle risk factor modification and grew out of North American and Northern European initiatives in the 1970s and 1980s (Farquhar *et al.*, 1990; Nutbeam *et al.*, 1990). In Ireland, we had the Kilkenny Health Project which ran from 1985 to 1991 (Shelley *et al.*, 1995). While virtually everyone has agreed by now on the shortcomings of the first generation community programs in health promotion, the explanations are different. The traditional objective is that the project acts as a focus which is supported by groups or opinion leaders within the community, and which works in the context of the social, cultural and physical environment. Supportive changes of varying kinds are instigated with a view to reaching individuals who accordingly should alter behaviour; this would have an impact on risk factors initially and ultimately on disease specific morbidity and mortality targets. By any standards, this is a highly complex undertaking which stretches the skills of the randomised control trial to its limit since the achievement of the outcome measure changes are so far removed from the complex process involved (Holman, 1997). The clinical experimental model was simply never envisaged for such tasks. Meanwhile the barrage of debate continues (Kelleher, 1992, 1995). Each time a study is reported we are required to re-visit a series of arguments along each step and the outcome is judged according to the position of the critic. If for instance you do not believe that serum cholesterol level (Skrabanek, 1992) can be altered significantly by dietary fat modification across programs, then a program that fails to reduce heart disease will be judged to have failed for this reason, though the explanation may lie elsewhere. Increasingly, the development of evidence-based medicine (Cochrane, 1972) has emphasised the importance of the randomised control trial model, but for reasons of feasibility, we have seen this is often not possible in a community-level situation. Again, as in other settings even the traditional interventions are over pessimistically interpreted. Despite the fact that sophisticated formative evaluations may be on-going (Flora *et al.*, 1993), it is the summative evaluations that receive the scrutiny.

Just like many other projects, the Kilkenny Health Project (Shelley *et al.*, 1995) showed beneficial risk factor changes at follow-up compared with baseline in terms of the lifestyle risk factors targeted, so that there were falls in the systolic blood pressure, cholesterol and smoking practice. There were increases in the number of individuals who had measured their cholesterol in the last year, though there were trends towards gains in obesity. The reference county, Offaly, did as well in most parameters measured with the exception of obesity, where the rates were much higher, and reported measure of cholesterol in the last year, which was also less frequent. It is quite clear that the social trends which influence both the establishment of such projects and the lifestyle behaviours in such populations, are at the very least occurring in parallel (Vartiainen *et al.*, 1994). While we cannot conclude with certainty that intervention projects *per se* influence the changes in the outcome risk factors we cannot refute it conclusively either. Nor does this mean that the investment in the process of such projects has not raised awareness, which would have long-term gains in relation to health behaviours, or that it is not having effects in terms of community participation or personal skills development that could be investments for the future. To answer these questions we need good measures of community dynamics, which is where the present day health promotion approach comes in. As a small example for instance, in the Kilkenny Health Project, within the reference county, Offaly, only about a third of people had reported such a cholesterol check as against over half in the Kilkenny area, but there was also a clear class gradient in Offaly, though not in Kilkenny (Kilkenny Health Project, 1995). It is possible that the project achieved better penetration for precisely those groups who most need contact and support whereas the more general hit and miss mass media educational approach to health matters which seems to be influential in Offaly was best taken up by middle-class people. Closer evaluation of these kind of questions will be important in the future.

REASONS FOR SETTING EFFECTS IN PROJECTS

So what can go wrong with an intervention project? First, it may simply not work. That's life and it does happen. However there are other explanations; it is also possible that the effect is small and therefore not sufficient to justify the approach at the expense of another kind of intervention and this is a major policy decision issue which I have referred to above. For the most part, however, the analysts are content to recommend social change policies as an alternative, rather than actually providing data which compare one kind of approach with another. Why for instance have we not focused more on passive versus active strategies, or designs which take account of both? Undoubtedly the logistical issues are complex, and very few countries have the resources to mount such trials that demand complex considerations of sample size and design at a quantitative level. To date, the disappointment of the existing trial data has mitigated against this.

The timescale may have been inappropriate in that it was too short for the level of anticipated achievement. This too is a resource issue. It is possible too that the comparison is invalid and not just because of contamination of one area by another. For the most part, quasi-experimental studies suffer from the fact that the reference areas do not stay the same over time, for reasons that are often confounding in nature. During the period of the Kilkenny Health Project for instance, butter consumption in Ireland plummeted (Friel and Nolan, 1996), most probably for a mixture of reasons, which included the huge supply of spread alternatives by co-operative creamery companies in the country. Finally, there is the possibility that the intervention is insufficient or inappropriate, and for the most part, the major studies reported today have focused on individual lifestyle change to the exclusion of a comprehensive account of other socio-cultural factors at play. We simply have not seen yet the kind of health promotion studies in practice that our theoretical thinking dictates.

What is normally concluded about intervention outcomes however runs something like this; that it does not work and the rest are just excuses. The traditional public health conclusion is that we should forget the individualistic educational approach and advocate social reform. There is no consensus on what this means; for some it may be as limited as the implementation of anti-tobacco regulations in public places, for others it is an assertion of the need for political change in society (Davey-Smith and Dorling, 1996). The health education conclusion, taken up more recently by the health promotion movement, is to forget the reductionist biomedical approach, because the methodologies are presently inadequate in any case, and the interventions for the most part have been unsubtle or short term. Such an approach would demand adequate personal and social development goals and resources for change that are culturally sympathetic. In some ways these positions are not all that far apart, particularly if both sides can see the positive elements in the existing intervention data and resist the impulse to throw the baby out with the bath water. Sadly, the policy-makers' conclusion overall in most countries is more pragmatic than either group and amounts to forgetting the whole thing and maintaining the status quo. Until we have a considerably more sophisticated inter-disciplinary interchange which is informed by the overriding need to effect health gain for populations, we are likely to see that the people with the power to make large-scale social reform in our societies will ignore the various researchers of different disciplines who manifestly cannot agree with each other. It is for this reason that the health promotion movement could have a vital role to play in the next few decades and why we need both a theoretical base and code of practice for setting and implementing standards.

CONCLUSIONS

While the period since the 1980s has provided a coherent political rhetoric and framework for health promotion (Nutbeam, 1997; WHO, 1986, 1988, 1991), we are without as yet, much of the precise information for operational quality assurance guidelines, but with broad scale evidence to support these kinds of conclusions. The strong case for health promotion derived from evidence about determinants of ill health, but the evidence on how to effect positive change has been more complicated. An adequately resourced, equitable and accessible education system that fosters knowledge, attitudes and life skills is a conclusion supported by education research over literally thousands of years. Its application to health promotion theory and practice has been indirect and the demonstration projects in train need to provide conclusions. An economy that delivers equitable standards of living and employment should in theory remove the inequities seen in health status within and between countries, but this is a political dimension which to date has not been analysed closely by the health promotion movement. The great political theories of the last two hundred years were not directly concerned with health status or with its measurement as an outcome; perhaps we should examine the issue more explicitly than we have to date. The Universal Declaration of Human Rights states that everyone has the right to a standard of living adequate for health and well-being (National Co-ordination Committee for UDHR 60; 1997). While we may believe that participative democracy is a civil or even a human right, in what way have we presented the evidence that it is a necessary prerequisite for health? A public policy system that regulates against hazards to human health and affords the individual choice and control in daily life, appears to be the area in which there is most potential agreement on all sides, and is informed by at least two centuries of such movements in developed countries. To date, however, across different countries, the expenditure in relation to such activities has been various both in relative and absolute terms.

At advocacy level, we may be left with a global aspiration to continue spending in relation to education, health and social welfare at the expense of health demoting activities; this is where work by people like Nancy Milio is so important in that it advocates real reforms in a practical and systematic way using the food chain as an example to promote nutritional health (Milio, 1986). There is increasing evidence that community intervention projects judged by criteria of enablement do show effects (Gillies, 1998) and we must be scrupulous in how these data are presented for the attention of policy-makers. Undoubtedly, the dominance of the reductionist scientific paradigm of the developed world has had significant influence on how we think about and evaluate health promotion programs. Scientific scepticism should not be the same as social conservatism, though neither a conservative nor a radical position has any place by itself in this debate. Rose (1992) pointed up the difference between decision-making at policy level and medical science, by reminding us that we can never be certain of anything, and that certainty is not a prerequisite for action. A sick person, he said, can expect from the physician only reasonable confidence that the diagnosis is right, and the treatment is likely to do more good, than harm. Preventive medicine should be judged in the same way, as indeed should health promotion. Like many before him, he advocated public policy structures that recognised the health demoting aspects of certain factors, and the health promoting aspects of others. But in our current market-based economy systems in the developed world, such regulations and controls are distasteful to many and come under increasing social pressure. Advocacy in this situation therefore can and should be informed by evidence. For the future, we continue to need a strong public health system, which advises on need and service/policy direction, and health promotion increasingly will be a 'how to' service which advises on effective and appropriate intervention at individual and policy level and which focuses on processes as much as outcome.

SUMMARY

It is clear that the settings-based movement evolved from a distillation of various disciplinary ideas. Such interventions must be seen in the context of wider public policy, and there is, at the moment, some pressure on the health promotion movement to prove, from a theoretical perspective, how such settings programs should work in practice. There may be a danger in the health promotion movement of attempting to evolve such theories without reference to much older and better established social science and biomedical disciplines. There are clearly social class and gender interactions in all settings-based situations, and we are only on the brink of understanding and refining these processes, though we do appear to be making some progress.

In the meantime, there is more evidence from schools, workplace and primary care settings of interventions' success, even using more traditional approaches, than is normally credited, and we need more dissemination of studies of good practice, and more discussion on appropriate intervention methodologies. The evaluative data may be over pessimistic, because of a self-imposed limitation in focus to biomedical outcomes for the most part, without a true acknowledgement of the complexity of showing such changes. This may be short changing the health promotion movement, and gives succour to critics who have no intention of altering the social status quo in terms of health determinants. If passive rather than individual based strategies are to be advocated, then opportunity cost data need to be produced to quantify what this would mean in a wider economic analysis of health promotion than we have seen to date. One valuable contribution of the modern health promotion movement has been to stress the diversity of means by which societies and individuals in society are empowered. This is the heart of the matter and the challenge for us all. There is no evidence to show that what appears intuitively sensible should not be advocated more widely in pilot or dissemination strategies, but is clear that more multi-discipline collaboration on appropriate methodologies will be needed to evaluate long-term gain in order to develop appropriate quality indicators.

Note

This chapter is based on a presentation to the first Summer School in Health Promotion held at University College Galway in July 1997. I would like to thank my colleagues at the Centre for Health Promotion Studies for the work which has contributed to this chapter, particularly Ms Saoirse Nic Gabhainn, Dr Ann Hope and Dr Una Fallon. Finally, my thanks to the ever patient Claire Mitchell for her help in preparing the manuscript.

References

Anderson, D.R. and Staufacker, M.J. (1996). The impact of worksite based health risk appraisal on health related outcomes: a review of the literature. *American Journal of Health Promotion* 10: 499–508.

Antonovsky, A. (1993). The sense of coherence as a determinant of health. In Beattie *et al.* (eds) *Health and Wellbeing: a Reader.* London: Macmillan Press Ltd: 202–15.

Antonovsky, A. (1996). The salutogenic model as theory to guide health promotion. *Health Promotion International* 11: 11–19.

Barker, D.J.P. and Osmond, C. (1986). Infant mortality, childhood nutrition and ischaemic heart disease in England and Wales. *Lancet* 1: 1,077–81.

Baxter, T., Milner, P., Wilson, K., Leaf, M., Nicholl, J., Freeman, J. and Cooper N. (1997). A cost effective community based heart health promotion project in England: prospective comparative study. *British Medical Journal* 315: 582–5.

Bobak, M. and Marmot, M.G. (1995). East/West mortality divide and its potential explanations: proposed research agenda. *British Medical Journal* 312: 421–5.

Booth, M.L. and Samdai, O. (1997). Health promoting schools in Australia: models and measurements. *Australian and New Zealand Journal of Public Health* 21: 365–71.

Bosma, H., Marmot, M.G., Hemingway, H., Nicholson, A.C., Brunner, E. and Stansfeld, S.A. (1997). Low job control and risk of CHD in Whitehall II (prospective cohort study). *British Medical Journal* 314: 558–65.

Bunker, J.P., Stansfeld, S. and Potter, J. (1996). Freedom, responsibility and health. *British Medical Journal* 313: 1,582–5.

Bygren, L.O., Benson Konlaan, B. and Johansson, S.E. (1996). Attendance at cultural events, reading books or periodicals, and making music or singing in a choir as determinants of survival: Swedish intervention survey of living conditions. *British Medical Journal* 313: 1,577–80.

Cainan, M., Boulton, M. and Williams, A. (1986). Health education and general practitioners: a critical appraisal. In Rodmell, S. and Watt, A. (eds) *The Politics of Heath Education: Raising the Issues.* London: Routledge & Kegan Paul: 183–204.

Chu, C., Driscoll, T. and Dwyer S. (1997). The health promoting workplace: an integrative perspective. *Australian and New Zealand Journal of Public Health* 2: 377–86.

Cochrane, A.L. (1972). *Effectiveness and Efficiency: Random Reflection on Health Services*. London: Nuffield Provincial Hospitals Trust.

Commit Research Group (1995). Community intervention trial for smoking cessation (COMMIT) II: changes in adult smoking prevalence. *American Journal of Public Health* 85: 193–200.

Davey-Smith, G. and Dorling, D. (1996). 'I'm all right John': voting patterns and mortality in England and Wales 1981–92. *British Medical Journal* 313: 1,573–7.

Davey-Smith, G. and Egger, M. (1996). Commentary: understanding it all – health, meta theories and mortality trends. *British Medical Journal* 313: 1,584–5.

Davey-Smith, G. and Egger, M. (1997). Changes in population distribution of sense of coherence do not explain changes in overall mortality. *British Medical Journal* 315: 490.

Davey-Smith, G., Hart, C., Blane, D., Gillis, C. and Hawthorne, V. (1997). Life time socio-economic position and mortality: prospective observational study. *British Medical Journal* 314: 547–52.

Davies, J.B. (1996). Health research: need for a methodological revolution. *Health Education Research: Theory and Practice* 11, i–iv.

Dean, K. (1996). Using theory to guide policy relevant health promotion research. *Health Promotion International* 11: 19–27.

Deccache, A. (1997). Evaluating quality and effectiveness: public health and social science approaches and methods (summary). *Promotion and Education* 4: 14–15.

Department of Health (1994). *Shaping a Healthier Future: A Strategy for Effective Healthcare in the 1990s*. Dublin: Department of Health.

Department of Health (1995). *A Health Promoting Strategy*. Dublin: Department of Health.

Ebrahim, S. and Davey-Smith, G. (1997). Systematic review of randomised controlled trials of multiple risk factor interventions for preventing coronary heart disease. *British Medical Journal* 314: 1,666–74.

Eddy, J.M., Fitzhugh, E.C., Wojtowicz, G.G. and Wang, M.Q. (1997). The effect of worksite based safety belt programs: a review of the literature. *American Journal of Health Promotion*, 11: 281–90.

Eickhoff-Shemek, and Ryan, K.F. (1995). A comparison of Omaha worksite health promotion activities to the 1992 National Survey with a special perspective on program intervention. *American Journal of Health Promotion* 10: 132–40.

Family Heart Study Group (1994). Randomised controlled trial evaluating cardiovascular screening and intervention in general practice: principal results of British Family Heart Study. *British Medical Journal* 308: 313–20.

Farquhar, J.W., Fortman, S.P., Flora, J.A., Taylor, C.B., Haskell, W.L., Williams, P.T., MacCoby, N. and Wood, P.D. (1990). Stanford Five City Project: effects of community wide education on cardiovascular disease risk factors. *Journal of the American Medical Association* 264: 359–65.

Fielding, J.R. (1996). Getting smarter and maybe wiser. *Health Promotion* 1: 109–12.

Fleming, S., Kelleher, C. and O'Connor, M. (1997). Eating patterns and factors influencing likely change in the workplace in Ireland. *Health Promotion International* 12: 187–96.

Flora, J.A., Lefebvre, R.C., Murray, D.A., Stone, E.J., Assaf, A., Mittelmark, M.B. and Finnegan, J.R. (1993). A community education monitoring system: methods from the Stanford FWC City project, Minnesota Heart Health Program and the Pawtucket Heart Health Program. *Health Education Research: Theory and Practice*: 81–95.

Friel, S. and Nolan, G. (1996). *Changes in the Food Chain since the Time of the Great Irish Famine*. Galway: National Nutrition Surveillance Centre, University College Galway.

Gillies, P. (1998). The effectiveness of alliances or partnerships for health promotion. *Health Promotion International* 13: 99–121.

Glanz, K., Sorenson, G. and Farmer, A. (1996). The health impact of worksite nutrition and cholesterol intervention programs. *American Journal of Health Promotion* 10: 453–71.

Goetzel, R., Kahr, T.Y., Aldana, S.G. and Kenny, G.M. (1996). An evaluation of Duke University's live for life health promotion program and its impact on employee health. *American Journal of Health Promotion* 10: 340–3.

Graham, H. and Hunt, S. (1994). Women's smoking and measures of women's socio-economic status in the United Kingdom. *Health Promotion International*: 81–9.

Green, L.W., Richard, L. and Potvin, L. (1996). Ecological foundations of health promotion. *Health Promotion* 16: 270–82.

Hawks, S.R., Hull, M.L., Thalman, R.L. and Richins, P.M. (1995). Review of spiritual health promotion: definition, role and intervention strategies in health promotion. *American Journal of Health Promotion* 9, 371–8.

Health Promoting School (1997). *A Challenge in Education, Health and Democracy*. Abstracts of proceedings of 1st conference of the European Network of Health Promoting Schools. Greece: Thessalonika, May.

Heaney, C.A. and Goetzel, R.Z. (1997). A review of health related outcomes of multi-component worksite health promotion programs. *American Journal of Health Promotion* 11: 290–307.

Hennrikus, D.J. and Jeffery, R.W. (1997). Worksite intervention for weight control: a review of the literature. *American Journal of Health Promotion* 10: 471–99.

Holman, C.D.A.J. (1997). Measuring the occurrence of health promoting interactions with the environment. *Australian and New Zealand Journal of Public Health* 21: 360–5.

Hope, A. and Kelleher C.C. (1995). *Health at Work: Lifestyle and Cancer: a Health Promotion Program in the Workplace*. Galway: Centre for Health Promotion Studies, University College Galway.

Hope, A., Kelleher, C.C. and O'Connor, M. (1997). Lifestyle practices and the health promoting environment of hospital nurses. *Journal of Advanced Nursing* 28.

Kelleher, C.C. (1991). Promoting health in young people. *Irish Medical Journal* 84: 81–3.

Kelleher, C.C. (1992). Promoting health. *Irish Medical Journal* 85: 75–6.

Kelleher, C.C. (1995). Health promotion: shades of Lewis Carroll. *Journal of Epidemiology and Community Health* 49: 1–4.

Kelleher, C.C. (1996). Education and training in health promotion: theory and methods. *Health Promotion International* 11: 47–55.

Kelleher, C.C. and Dineen, B. (1993). Health promotion in schools. *British Medical Journal* 306: 517.

Kickbusch, I. (1996). New players for a new era: how up to date is health promotion. *Health Promotion International* 11: 259–63.

Kickbusch, I. (1997). Health promoting environments: the next steps. *Australian and New Zealand Journal of Public Health* 21: 431–4.

Kilkenny Health Project (1995). *Final Report*. Dublin: Department of Health.

Labonte, R. (1989). Community health promotion strategies. In C.J. Martin and D.V. McQueen (eds) *Readings for a New Public Health*. Edinburgh: Edinburgh University Press: 235–49.

Love, M.B., Davili, G.W. and Thurman, O.C. (1996). Normative beliefs of health behaviour professionals regarding the psychosocial and environmental factors that influence health behaviour change related to smoking cessation, regular exercise and weight loss. *American Journal of Health Promotion* 10: 371–80.

Lynch, P. (1995). Adolescent smoking – an alternative perspective using personal construct theory. *Health Education Research: Theory and Practice* 10: 95–106.

MacDonald, G. (1997). Quality indicators and health promotion effectiveness. *Promotion and Education* 4: 5–8.

McLeroy, K.R., Steckler, A.B., Simon, S., Morton, B., Goodman, R.M., Gottlieb, N. and

Burdine, J.N. (1993). Social science theory in health education: time for a new model. *Health Education Research: Theory and Practice* 8: 305–13.

McQueen, D. (1996). The search for theory in health behaviour and health promotion. *Health Promotion International* 11: 27–33.

Milio, N. (1986). *Promoting Health through Public Policy*. Ottawa: Canadian Public Health Association.

Murphy, L.R. (1996). Stress management in work settings: a critical review of the health effects. *American Journal of Health Promotion* 11: 136–50.

National Co-ordination Committee for UDHR 60 (1997). *Drafting and Adoption: The Universal Declaration of Human Rights*. Washington: Franklin and Eleanor Roosevelt Institute.

Nic Gabhainn, S. and Kelleher, C.C. (1995). *Life Skills for Health Promotion: The Evaluation of the North Western Health Board's Health Education Programme*. Galway: Centre for Health Promotion Studies, University College Galway.

Nic Gabhainn, S. and Kelleher, C.C. (1996). Qualitative perspectives on coronary heart disease: a challenge to the applicability of models of health behaviour? Proceedings of the Annual Conference of the European Health Psychology Society. Dublin. September.

Nic Gabhainn, S. and Kelleher, C.C. (1997). *Irish Network of Health Promoting Schools*. Galway: Centre for Health Promotion Studies, University College Galway.

Nutbeam, D. (1996). Healthy islands – a truly ecological model of health promotion. *Health Promotion International* 11: 263–5.

Nutbeam, D. (1997). (Editorial) Creating health promoting environments: overcoming barriers to action. *Australian and New Zealand Journal of Public Health* 21: 355–60.

Nutbeam, D. and Aaro, L.E. (1991). Smoking and pupil attitudes towards school: the implications for health education with young people. Results from the WHO study of health behaviour among school children. *Health Education Research: Theory and Practice* 6: 415–21.

Nutbeam, D., Macaskill, P., Smith, C., Simpson, J. and Catford, J.C. (1993). Evaluation of two school smoking education programs under normal classroom conditions. *British Medical Journal* 306: 102–7.

Nutbeam, D., Smith, C., Murphy, S. and Catford J. (1990). Maintaining evaluation designs in long term community based health promotion programs: Heartbeat Wales study. *Journal of Epidemiology and Community Health* 47: 127–33.

O'Connor, E.A., Friel, S. and Kelleher, C.C. (1997). Fashion consciousness as a social influence on lifestyle behaviour in young Irish adults. *Health Promotion International* 12: 135–41.

O'Donnell, M., Fallon, U. and Kelleher, C.C. (1997). Process evaluation of a health promotion education resource material for children: Galway Health Project. Proceedings of the Nutrition Society, Irish Section, Dublin, 57; 23A.

O'Donnell, M. (1996) (Editorial). *American Journal of Health Promotion* 10: 424.

Ovretveit, J. (1996). Quality in health promotion. *Health Promotion International* 11: 55–63.

Parson, C., Stears, D., Thomas, C., Thomas, L. and Holland, J. (1997). *The implications of ENHPS (European Network of Health Promoting Schools) in different national contexts*. Canterbury: Centre for Health Education and Research, Canterbury Christ Church College.

Pelletier, K.R. (1996). A review and analysis of the health and cost effective outcome studies of comprehensive health promotion and disease prevention programs at the worksite: 1993–1995 update. *American Journal of Health Promotion* 10, 380–9.

Roman, P.H. and Blum, T. C. (1996). Alcohol: a review of the impact of worksite interventions on health and behavioural outcomes. *American Journal of Health Promotion* 11: 136–50.

Rootman, I. (1997). Continuous quality improvement in health promotion: some preliminary thoughts from Canada. *Promotion and Education* 4: 23–5.

Rose, G. (1992). *The Strategy of Preventive Medicine*. Oxford: Oxford Medical Publications, Oxford University Press.

Russell, M.A.H., Wilson, C., Taylor, C. and Baker, C.D. (1979). Effects of general practitioners' advice against smoking. *British Medical Journal* 231–5.

Saan, H. (1997). Quality revisited. *Promotion and Education* 4: 34–5.

Shelley, E., Daly, L., Collins, C., Christie, M., Conroy, R., Gibney, M., Hickey, N., Kelleher, C., Kilcoyne, D., Lee, P., Mulcahy, R., Murray, P., O'Dwyer, T., Radic, A. and Graham, I. (1995). Cardiovascular risk factor changes in the Kilkenny Health Project: a community health promotion program. *European Heart Journal* 16: 752–60.

Shephard, R. J. (1996). Worksite fitness and exercise programs: a review of methodology and health impact. *American Journal of Health Promotion* 10: 436–53.

Siegrist, J. (1993). Sense of coherence and sociology of emotions. *Social Science and Medicine* 37: 978–9.

Skrabanek, P. (1992). Promoting health. *Irish Medical Journal* 85: 75.

Sorensen, G., Stoddard, A., Hammond, K., Herbert, J.R., Spitz Avrunin, J. and Ockene, J. K. (1996). Double jeopardy: workplace hazards and behavioural risks for craftspersons and labourers. *American Journal of Health Promotion* 10: 355–64.

Squires, N. and Strobl, J. (1997). *Healthy Prisons: a Vision for the Future*. Liverpool: Report of 1st International Conference on Healthy Prisons, University of Liverpool.

Susser, M. (1995) (Editorial) The tribulations of trials – intervention in communities. *American Journal of Public Health* 85: 156–8.

Terborg, J.R., Hibbard, J. and Glasgow, R.E. (1995). Behaviour change at the worksite: does social support make a difference? *American Journal of Health Promotion* 10: 125–32.

Tones, K. (1997). Beyond the randomised controlled trial: a case for 'judicial review'. *Health Education Research: Theory and Practice* 12: i–iv.

Vartiainen, E., Puska, P., Pekkanen, J., Tuomilemto, J. and Jousilamti, P. (1994). Changes in risk factors explain changes in mortality from ischaemic heart disease in Finland. *British Medical Journal* 309: 23–8.

Wilson, M.G., Hocman, P.B. and Hammock, A. (1996a). A comprehensive review of the effects of worksite health promotion on health related outcomes. *American Journal of Health Promotion* 10: 429–36.

Wilson, M.G., Jorgensen, C. and Cole, G. (1996b). The health effects of worksite HIV/AIDS interventions: a review of the research literature. *American Journal of Health Promotion* 11: 150.

World Health Organization (1986). *The Ottawa Charter on Health Promotion*. Ottawa: Canadian Public Health Association.

World Health Organization (1988). *Healthy Public Policy. Adelaide Recommendations*. WHO. Geneva: Health Education and Health Promotion Unit.

World Health Organization (1991). *Supportive Environments for Health. The Sundsvall Statement*. WHO. Geneva: Health Education and Health Promotion Unit.

Ziglio, E. (1997). How to move towards evidence-based health promotion interventions. *Promotion and Education* 4: 29–33.

Chapter 4

Measuring effectiveness in community-based health promotion

Frances Baum

INTRODUCTION

Health promotion experience since the 1970s has produced convincing evidence that campaigns, implemented across large populations, designed to persuade people to change their behaviour are not overly successful. In the light of these findings health promoters are turning more and more to working with people in their local communities and other settings and using strategies derived from community development in efforts to improve health status. This approach is evident in the work of community health centres, Healthy Cities initiatives and the 'settings approach' in schools and workplaces, for instance. The approach rests on a view of health as a reflection of the social, economic and environmental circumstances of individuals and their communities. It draws on the idea that power and control have a significant impact on health and so 'empowerment' and participation are central concepts to community-based health promotion initiatives.

Much of the appeal of the behavioural and lifestyle interventions so popular in the 1970s and 1980s was because they could be evaluated by drawing on the techniques of conventional biomedical science. While these scientific techniques had to be adapted to the needs of community-based trials, the basic logic underlying them was used as the justification of the evaluation of many of the large lifestyle campaigns such as the 'Mr Fit' programme (Winklestein and Marmot, 1981), the North Karelia project in Finland (Puska *et al.*, 1985) and the Stanford Five City project (Farquhar, 1984). Community-based health promotion, using community development strategies, can not easily be adapted to the biomedical paradigm and consequently poses challenges for evaluators accustomed to those methodologies. This chapter will describe the features of community-based health promotion and consider the ways in which they can be evaluated and issues raised by the evaluation process.

WHAT IS COMMUNITY-BASED HEALTH PROMOTION?

Community based health promotion in this chapter is taken to mean activities within communities designed to promote health in a manner consistent with the principles espoused in the Ottawa Charter (WHO, 1986). Health promotion, according to the Ottawa Charter, is the process of 'enabling people to increase control over, and to improve, their health'. Community-based health promotion aims to encourage empowerment amongst the community and, to this end, is based on a model of professional practice which stresses partnership rather than professional dominance. Community development is a key strategy. Its practice draws heavily on the work of Freire (1972) who advocated education for liberation which followed these stages:

- reflection on peoples' lived reality;
- analysis and collective identification of the root cause of that reality;
- examination of their implication;
- development of a plan of action to bring about change.

In this process professionals and community people should ideally meet as equals and develop a dialogue based on trust. The aim of the process is critical consciousness raising.

The benefits of basing health promotion activity in community settings and using community development strategies has received increasing recognition. The characteristics of the approach have been elaborated by a number of authors (Fry 1989; Baum *et al.*, 1992; Sanderson and Alexander, 1995; Tesoriero, 1995; Labonte, 1992; Legge *et al.*, 1996) and the summary of main features of community-based health promotion in Box 1 are based on a synthesis of this work.

The understanding of health underlying community-based health promotion is based on a socio-environmental approach which encompasses medical, behavioural and community development strategies (Labonte, 1992). It recognises the different levels of power that groups within society hold and that power levels can influence the ability of individuals to promote their own health. Ideally, community-based health promotion initiatives are derived from issues identified from members of the community, rather than by professional health workers. Community members are also seen as integral to the planning, implementation and evaluation of the initiatives.

The 'community' may be a geographic community but can also refer to a community of interest such as people with a particular health issue or from a particular ethnic group. The term community is sometimes interpreted to include the gender, ethnicity, class and age diversities typical of contemporary societies. The interpretation of 'community' in discussions of community-based health promotion varies in its degree of sophistication. Some policy statements treat the term uncritically and use 'community' to evoke warm, nostalgic notions of a by-gone age and do not acknowledge the power dimensions, conflicts and diversity that typify most communities. Other commentators are far more analytical and point out that 'community' is a complex term which means different things to different groups and often masks considerable tensions, inequities and diversity (see for example Petersen and Lupton, 1996).

Box 1
Main features of community-based health promotion

Principles

- uses a socio-environmental approach to health promotion which encompasses medical, behavioural and community development strategies;
- based on a recognition of the importance of power differentials in determining health outcomes and the abilities of groups to promote their own health;
- recognises the diversity of communities and the particular needs of sub-groups within a defined area, in terms of variables such as of gender, ethnicity, class and age;
- concerned with achieving equitable health outcomes;
- is informed and strengthened by the participation of local people in management, programme planning, implementation and evaluation.

Style of practice

- focuses on the health of the people in a defined geographic area or community of interest;
- community members define the issues on which the health promotion effort focuses;
- development, through a partnership between community members and professionals, of a comprehensive knowledge of local people, their environment and needs;
- uses this knowledge to identify and analyse local health issues, and to develop and implement initiatives;
- rests on models of professional practice which stress partnerships with communities and strives to overcome professional hegemony;
- involves advocacy and the provision of a public voice for the health of the local community;
- main strategies are based on community development practice.

The approach is not just concerned with promoting health *per se*, but also with a focus on improving the health of the least healthy (such as indigenous peoples in Australia). The Ottawa Charter for Health Promotion stresses the importance of countries working towards greater equity between different groups in society. Health promotion, based on strategies designed to achieve behavioural change alone, may well increase health inequities because those people whose living conditions (housing, income, employment, for instance) are relatively good are the most likely to be able to incorporate lifestyle changes into their lives. Only approaches which tackle the underlying conditions of illness will have much impact on poverty.

One of the challenges community-based health promotion poses for evaluation is that it is based on concepts and theories that are complex and, in some cases, disputed. This is particularly the case for community development practice and the theories underlying it, such as empowerment and participation. Community development has been growing in both popularity and credibility in a number of areas, including public health. This has happened most noticeably through the work of development agencies in developing countries. International agencies such as the World Bank, United Nations Development Program (UNDP) and many non-government organisations have seen community development as the answer to improving the living conditions of the world's poorest people.

Community development has also been used in developed countries. The strategy has been used by social workers since the 1970s. Many urban renewal projects in the United Kingdom, for instance, have used these strategies. In Australia community development has been used as a strategy throughout the post-Second World War period. Agriculture projects used it extensively in the 1940s and 1950s (Dixon, 1989). But it was under the Whitlam Labor Government (1973–75) that community development flourished. Many of its programmes used strategies based on community development. Since that time community development as a health promotion strategy has been a common method of working used by community health centres, particularly in the States of Victoria (CDIH, 1988; Jackson *et al.*, 1989) and South Australia (Tesoriero, 1995). Its practice within state-funded services has always been problematic. One reason for this is that workers using community development strategies will often find themselves working on issues that bring them into conflict with the government department that funds them (Baum, Sanderson and Jolley, 1997).

Mayo and Craig (1995) pose the question of whether the use of community development is always used as a tool of democratic transformation or whether, for agencies such as the World Bank, it serves as the 'human face of structural adjustment'. It is quite likely that the World Bank uses terms such as *empowerment* quite differently to a progressive NGO such as Community Aid Abroad. The same is true of the use of the terms within developed countries. Government departments are likely to use terms such as *empowerment* in a quite rhetoric way, whereas workers in a community health centre may be engaged in real attempts to work with disempowered people so that they can exercise a little more power in their lives. Despite these reservations and, even in the face of problematic questions such as this, Mayo and Craig (1995) recognise that community development and participation are still vital. They see these strategies being increasingly advocated in both the North and the South in 'the context of increasing poverty, polarisation and social exclusion' (p. 3). There has been much thinking about its practice and theory in relation to public health (see, for example, CDIH, 1988; Baum, 1988; Dixon, 1989; McWalters *et al.*, 1989; Dwyer, 1989; Wass, 1994; Labonte, 1992; Legge *et al.*, 1996). This literature makes it clear that the practice of community development is theoretically challenging. These challenges are just as real to evaluators as to practitioners.

EVALUATION

This section begins with a description of a framework within which evaluation can be structured. It then discusses the value of participatory approaches to evaluation. Issues associated with conducting and managing the evaluation are then considered. The processes, objectives, outcomes and key methods of evaluation are then described. Finally, interpretation and reporting are discussed.

Evaluation framework

The stages of an evaluation fit into the following categories: assessing the preconditions that shaped the project; describing how the project started out; describing the implementation and then assessing the value of the project's processes and outcomes. Key questions for each of these stages are provided in Box 2.

One factor which makes evaluation easier is if the idea and acceptance of evaluation has been built into the initiative early on in its life. This may not always happen as community projects may arise spontaneously and organically rather than as 'planned' and predestined. Nonetheless, the sooner evaluation can be incorporated the more useful it is for development and the more accurately it will be able to report on the initiative.

Community-based health promotion with the characteristics described in the previous section is based on the belief that participation is an essential element of a successful project. Consequently, evaluation practices should also develop participatory methodologies. In public health research generally it has been increasingly suggested that research should become less of an elitist endeavour and be more inclusive of the people being researched (see, for example, Wadsworth, 1984; Feuerstein, 1986; Raeburn, 1992; Baum, 1996; de Koning and Martin, 1996). In Australia indigenous people have become particularly sceptical of academic researchers in terms of the value of much research to them and the lack of control they have been able to exert over it (Colin and Garrow, 1996). See Kemmis and McTaggart (1988) for a summary of the method and Wadsworth (1991), de Koning and Martin (1996) and Kennedy (1995) for examples of the method applied to health.) Participatory action research (PAR) conceives of evaluation as a spiral process of planning, fieldwork, analysis, reflection and then a spiralling up to planning again. The spiral analogy is particularly suited to community-based health promotion because it captures its dynamic nature and incorporates the shifting and changing nature of this work.

The practice of action research in health promotion does present dilemmas. Boutilier *et al.* (1997) describe a number of these and argue that the perspectives of academic researchers, practitioners (managerial and frontline) and community members differ and argue that to be effective action research requires considerable negotiation and reflection on practice. They suggest (p.76) that key issues in

Box 2
Key questions for the evaluation of community-based health promotion

Preconditions
Description of the setting in which the initiative happened including history of community development action
Description of any activity related to the initiative being evaluated which had occurred before

Starting out
How did the initiative start?
Who defined the issues? How?
Who was involved?
What were the original objectives?
How long did the initiative take to get started?
What were the significant events?
What experience or theory suggested the initiative might achieve its aims?
How has the initiative been funded?

Implementing
Provide full description of what activities and processes the initiative has involved
What have been the main events?
Who has been involved?
What have their different expected outcomes been?
Has the involvement of different groups changed over time?

Assessment
What have been the achievements?
What have been the disappointments?
How can the achievements and disappointments be explained?
What strategies were most successful?
Which were not successful?
How do the participants perceive they have been changed by their involvement?
What have they learnt through their involvement?
What changes in the environment affected the initiative?
What lessons have been learnt?
How have the original objectives changed?
Did the outcomes fit with previous experience and theory?

the practice of what they describe as *community reflective action research* are those to do with whose knowledge is valued, who owns the research, why the research is being done and the importance of recognising the complementary skills of community members, researchers and practitioners. Community participation and control of research processes may lead to some conflicts with the demands of scientific rigour (Allison and Rootman, 1996) as community people are generally not experts in research or primarily interested in the validity of research. This tension should be addressed by evaluators so that ideally, evaluations are scientifically acceptable and ethically participatory!

The processes of negotiation involved in participatory action research make it a long and complicated process. This will often conflict with the needs of funding bodies which often require short and straightforward reports on progress. It is not easy to reconcile these conflicting demands.

Evaluations of community-based health promotion tend to vary in the degree of participation they involve. Some will be participatory throughout the entire research process (setting the research agenda, deciding on methods, collecting and analysing data and in reporting and applying findings). Others will involve participation in some aspects of these processes only. Evaluation may be conducted in a way that ensures people have some involvement and that their perspective is represented but will not involve them as equal partners. This may happen for a variety of reasons including requirements of funding bodies, the involvement of outside researchers, the evaluation is retrospective rather than prospective, or time constraints. Given the philosophy of community-based health promotion stresses the central importance of participation, evaluations should be as participatory as is feasible.

CONDUCTING AND MANAGING THE EVALUATION

Insider or outsider evaluation?

Evaluation can be conducted by the people responsible for the particular programme – an insider's evaluation. Alternatively it may be conducted by outsiders. There is no inherent benefit with either an insider or outsider evaluation, there are advantages and some drawbacks to both approaches (Feuerstein, 1986). The decision about which to choose will depend on the resources available to do the evaluation, the purpose of doing the evaluation, requirement of funding bodies, the stage of the intervention being evaluated. The important thing is that the choice should be thought through as part of the planning stage for the evaluation. In situations where the primary reason for the evaluation is developmental an internal evaluation may be preferable. In instances where the evaluation is being conducted primarily for external interests the evaluation may gain legitimacy by being external. Either way the evaluation should be as participatory as possible.

Appropriate timing for evaluation

The developmental nature of community development means that evaluation cannot happen in a short timeframe. Five years is realistic. A sustained effort is required to develop a group of people, for them to define their objectives, take action, learn from their mistakes and establish sufficient confidence in their ability to effect change. Funders often want evaluation results over a much shorter timeframe. Process information on the establishment of an initiative is likely to be the most important information in the shorter term. This information can be crucial to the development and refinement of the initiative and provide managers and funders with a clear idea of how the project is proceeding.

Resources

The scope and approach of any evaluation has to be tailored to the available resources. As a rough rule of thumb a community health promotion project should consider spending approximately 10 per cent of the cost of an intervention on evaluation. Managers and funders of community-based health promotion initiatives should ensure that resources are available to fund and support evaluation. In South Australia the South Australian Health Commission has, for more than a decade, funded the South Australia Community Health Research Unit. This unit provides evaluation advice to community health workers in the state, runs staff development sessions on evaluation and conducts specific evaluations. Such organisational support is crucial as it assists in creating a culture in which evaluation is valued.

Community health workers are often very action-orientated and may be reluctant to spend time on collecting data, documenting and producing reports. This is where a researcher working in partnership can be of great assistance to a community project. They can become the voice of a project and ensure its achievements and challenges are documented so that they can contribute to broader debates.

Evaluation skills

A good evaluator is likely to be a creative and lateral thinker and be able to assess the initiative they are evaluating within its local social and political context. The data will not speak for itself and needs to be interpreted through the perspective of the evaluator who can be greatly assisted in this process by discussing the findings with participants. The evaluator: 'assumes the position of being an orchestrator of opinion, an arranger of data, a summariser of what is commonly held, a collector of suggestions for change, a sharpener of policy alternatives' (Parlett, 1981, p. 234). If the evaluator is able to achieve this then evaluation can become part of the development process.

Ideally all health promotion and community development staff should have well-developed skills in evaluation. While this is sometimes the case, more commonly these skills are not strong or seen as a priority. A recent review of a national health promotion funding programme in South Australia (Baum *et al.*, 1997) and of the South Australian Primary Health Care Advancement

Program (SACHRU, 1997) reported that many of the project officers employed on the funded projects felt that they did not have sufficient evaluation skills. This had made evaluating their projects difficult even though some formal evaluation advice was organised for them. They also reported a 'fear of evaluation' that was exacerbated by the jargon of evaluation which makes it confusing for experts let alone those new to the endeavour.

Evaluating the organisational and funding context of community-based health promotion

Evaluation is, inevitably, a political process. Whoever conducts an evaluation cannot avoid being tied up with organisational politics and possibly broader political agendas. Inevitably community development in health projects involves a range of vested interests (Hunt, 1987; Marsden and Oakley, 1991). Professionals, funding bodies and community people will all have different perspectives and expectations of any particular intervention.

An evaluator should attempt to assess the politics of the setting of their evaluation and will have to keep a constant watch for the impact of political issues, as the evaluation proceeds. A good evaluation incorporates the complexities of any situation (Furler, 1979) but does not become so complex that its findings are too dense to be useful (Wadsworth, 1991).

Organisational context

An important aspect of the evaluation of community-based health promotion is consideration and assessment of the organisational setting of the community-based health promotion initiative. This setting shapes the potential of projects and can either help or hinder their progress.

The ultimate aim of community development in health is to empower people and their communities in such a way that individual and collective health status is improved. The evaluation and management of community development requires considerable flexibility. As a public health strategy it does not easily fit within rational planning, management and evaluation frameworks. The values base (specified in the previous section) of community development and the relinquishing of at least some control to the community means that public health organisations have to ensure that they develop management frameworks that support community development activity. Evaluation of projects should assess the degree to which the organisation supports community-based health promotion.

Funding context

The experiences of health promoters suggest that community development is often not understood and valued by health funding authorities. The work is often diffuse and it is hard to specify in advance exactly what form the initiative will take. Indeed, if it could be specified in advance then it almost certainly would not be community development. The process of working with communities is invariably messy and a lot less controllable than traditional health promotion which selected a target group and then delivered a pre-set programme. These latter approaches fit the rational planning frameworks preferred by most bureaucracies. Often a health authority may identify the local health problems to be connected with issues such as child health and parenting, older people, mental health and services for ethnic minorities. By contrast the community may identify quite different priorities such as developing anti-racist strategies within the health services and the community, building community health organisation, developing community and user representation in the health services, and raising awareness of health issues. In such situations the health worker will find themselves caught between the expectations of their employer and the accountability they owe to the community. To follow the community may mean risking their employment status; to meet the expectations of their employer would mean betraying the trust of the community and so undoing what is likely to have been a considerable amount of groundwork.

A further problem of community development, from the perspective of funding bodies, is the developmental and long-term nature of the work. Often health promotion projects using community development as their basis are funded only for a short period. In this time, in a disempowered and disadvantaged community it will often only be possible to establish legitimacy, gain trust and work out some priorities for action. If funding ceases at this point very little will have been gained. Much community development work has to be seen as an investment that to yield maximum rewards should take place over a long timescale. This is one reason why community health centres are well positioned to be the centre of community development in health activity. They will be known to the community and have developed trust. Activities will be able to build on each other and the community can develop a sense of ownership not just of particular initiatives but of the centre itself. They can help overcome the difficulties of short-term funding.

PROCESS, OBJECTIVES AND OUTCOMES

Process

Nearly all evaluations will be concerned with collecting information on and assessing both the process of implementing a community-based health promotion initiative and with the outcomes that have been achieved. Evaluating the process is crucial because this information is usually essential to determining why the particular outcomes were as they were. In effect, evaluation of process opens the project's black box and provides detailed insight into the operation and dynamics of the initiative. The developmental nature of most community-based health promotion makes this information vital to learning from the project and improving practice in the future. Timely process evaluation can identify ways in which an initiative could be improved and so play a part in achieving better outcomes.

Objectives

The specific objectives of a community development initiative can rarely be specified in advance. These depend on definition by the community and may take some time to evolve. They are also likely to shift and change as the context and participants change. The activities and objectives of most community-based health promotion change as they have successes and failures and so refocus on new activities as new opportunities and partnerships develop. These shifting objectives make it more difficult for evaluators but have to be incorporated within the evaluation if it is to do its job of describing and assessing the progress of the initiative thoroughly.

Outcomes

Defining and measuring outcomes in community-based health promotion is both difficult in itself and requires the recognition that the choice of outcome measure will depend on whose perspective is chosen. In evaluating community development different groups who are involved may not even agree on what the outcome of a project should be let alone whether or not it has been achieved (Hunt, 1987). Funding bodies, community people, community health workers, community health managers may all have different perceptions on what the crucial outcomes should be. The evaluation process needs to specify these differing interests in advance and then ensure that the evaluation pays attention to each of them. Obviously each group's values become crucial in this process.

It is recognised that while the rationale for community development programmes is the promotion of health, the immediate objectives relate more to empowerment and the creation of conditions that are likely to promote health (Baum, 1995; Legge *et al.*, 1996; Sheills and Hawe, 1996). Sheills and Hawe (1996) argue that evaluation of community development should ensure that it measures change at a community level and individual level. They suggest that communities are more than the sum of the individuals within them, and that this is a challenge to conventional research techniques which focus on individuals and the aggregate of individual change. They do not, however, provide specific guidance about exactly how community empowerment can be measured at a collective level. The question is, perhaps, most likely to be answered in the context of a specific project. Thus, as part of an evaluation, it is necessary to agree on what may be appropriate outcomes. A useful framework within which to do this is the following:

- Individual health status outcomes
- Community health status outcomes
- Changes in any of the conditions that shape the health of communities
- Increased capacities of:

    community members
    institutions
    professionals

Focusing on individual, community, institutional and professional change will assist in ensuring that an evaluation process does not make the mistake Sheills and Hawe (1996) caution against.

Changes in the conditions that create health and an increased capacity are probably the most likely outcomes from community development projects. Health status outcomes are unlikely to be able to be directly attributed to any particular community development activity because there will almost certainly be other factors which contribute to individual and community health status.

Different players in an evaluation may well expect different outcomes. One of the tasks of an evaluator is to determine what each group with an interest in the evaluation expects the outcomes of a particular exercise might be and (importantly) to monitor how these might change over the life of the initiative. Table 4.1 may be a useful tool in doing this. It is completed for a community action group established with support from a community development worker in a community health centre working to minimise environmental pollution from local industries in a working-class residential area. The group was active in an Australian state and one result of their activity was the establishment of a regional intersectoral committee to deal with environmental issues which involved community, industry and government.

Table 4.1 demonstrates that different players will have very different expectations from the same initiative. The Minister of Health, for example, is initially only interested in whether she can see a demonstrated impact on health status in the catchment area of the community health centre. By contrast the community members start off with the ambitious desire to stop all pollution. Two of the key players, the local industries and the Department of Economic Development, were not even involved at the outset but became so as the project progressed and their desired outcomes would then have to be incorporated as part of the evaluation, even though they were not involved initially. In this case it is clear that the outcome desired by the Department of Economic Development – not to have environmental concerns obstruct development projects in the region – was at odds with the aims of the residents and community development worker. Some of the original desired outcomes were not present at a later stage. Thus the manager of the community health centre who had originally hoped to be able to detect a reduction in asthma admissions at the local hospital came

Table 4.1 Example of a table to monitor changing expectations of key players in a community-based health promotion initiative

Key players	Initial expected outcomes	Revised expected outcomes
Community members	*Stop the pollution*	Gain skills in lobbying politicians and local industry leaders Reduce pollution Prevent new polluting industries setting up in the community Give a community voice to the local intersectoral environmental group
Community development worker	Ensure community involvement in the project Raise local awareness about the health effects of industrial pollution Have some effect on the practices of local industry	The group can operate effectively with less support from the centre than needed initially The people involved gain skills and knowledge that they can use more generally in their lives Local industry comes to see benefits of maintaining dialogue with community group
Manager of community health centre	The community health centre establishes a reputation as a place of best practice for community development in health *Less asthma admissions at local hospital*	Community health centre seen as central player in local intersectoral environmental forum involving community, industry, health and local government Community health centre seen as responsive to the needs of the local community
Health department funding the community health centre	The initiative is in line with service agreement It is value for money *The impact of the initiative on health outcomes in the area*	Model example of implementation of primary health care policy
State Minister for Health	*The impact of the initiative on health outcomes in the area*	Effective means of dealing with conflict over environmental issues in the region Potential to provide voter support
State Ministry of Economic Development	No involvement or expectations	Concerned the achievements of group do not interfere with economic development in the region
Local industry	No involvement or expectations	Able to communicate with the community group to prevent adverse publicity Means of industries appearing responsive to the concerns of community

Note: initial expected outcomes in italics are those that were dropped as the scheme progressed.

to appreciate that this was unlikely. A more useful and realistic outcome measure was the extent to which the community health centre came to be seen as a key player in intersectoral negotiations about environmental health issues. The use of such a table by evaluators can be a useful tool to display changing and conflicting objectives and so analyse the progress of the initiative.

Appropriate methods

Until recently, public health has been dominated by epidemiological research methods, which, in turn, are drawn from the practices of biomedical science. For epidemiology the gold standard has been the randomised control trial. The appeal of this method is that if the public health intervention group can be matched with a control group which does not experience the intervention then conclusions about causal attribution can be drawn. If this method were to be applied to community-based health promotion then the following three conditions would have to be met:

- The control community would have to be largely the same as one experiencing the intervention.
- The control community would have to have no health promotion intervention of its own.
- The external forces on the control and experimental communities would have to be very similar.

The organic, developmental and practical aspects of community-based health promotion make it impossible to meet these conditions.

The naturalistic setting of community development and its evolution mean that the idea of a control community is impractical. Even in health promotion programmes that are largely based on behaviour change goals, control communities are not as attractive a methodological solution as they might, at first, appear. Nutbeam *et al.* (1993), for instance, describe the experience of the Heartbeat Wales evaluators when they used a control area for their intervention area. The control area decided to adopt their own heart health programme and so was ineffective as a control. Additionally while communities may often be similar they are never going to be identical so their power to determine patterns of causality is reduced.

The activity in a community development initiative is essentially human-centred and about the interaction and relationships between people and between people and organisations and institutions. Evaluation methods have to be powerful enough to capture the subtleties and nuances of these relationships, to capture the dynamics and tease out the successes and failures and the likely reasons for them. Epidemiology aims to control variables so that predictions can be made. Inevitably it is reductionist in its attempt to achieve this. The focus is on measurement and description. By contrast the job of the evaluator in coming to understand community-based health promotion is on more open inquiry which aims at understanding the social processes that have occurred. This process of inquiry has more in common with constructivist approaches to inquiry which aim at reconstruction of previously held constructions (Lincoln, 1992). In this sense the evaluator is more of a storyteller, facilitator and interpreter than a manipulator and controller of events.

In seeking to understand and interpret an initiative, the evaluator is likely to draw on a range of methods that collect both qualitative and quantitative data. The scientific approach is to select those methods which provide the information necessary to provide an interpretation of the community initiative that will satisfy the needs of the key players. These methods must include those which enable description, interpretation and understanding. The methods must also be chosen to fit the available budget and the timescale available for the evaluation. They include focus group and individual interviews, self-completion surveys, participant observation, journals kept by project participants, analysis of community and organisational networks, records from official documents (including minutes and policies) and analysis of media coverage. A brief description of these methods and their likely use in community-based health promotion evaluation is provided below. Another method is the story dialogue technique (Labonte and Feather, 1996) described in Macdonald and Davies (in this volume).

Personal interviews

Detailed interviews can be an effective means of gaining insight into the dynamics of an initiative and the different assessment of it made by different people. In essence interviews are a form of discussion which aims to collect elucidating information. They can collect far more detailed information than is possible in a self-completion questionnaire. If a health promotion initiative has focused on a topic that is sensitive (for example, spouse abuse or child sexual abuse) then interviews are likely to be the preferred method of evaluation. They are, however, usually time-consuming to conduct and analyse. This has to be balanced against the very detailed information they provide. A number of texts provide detailed information on conducting these interviews (Spradley, 1979; Minichello *et al.*, 1990).

Focus group interviews

Focus groups usually involve conducting open-ended interviews with between five and ten people on an aspect of the project being evaluated. It has been claimed that these groups 'are not just a convenient way to accumulate the individual knowledge of their members. They give rise synergistically to insights and solutions that would not come about without them' (Brown *et al.*, 1989, p. 40). They are useful if the evaluator wants to provide participants with the opportunity to be wide-ranging in their comments about an initiative. The difficulties they pose are that a form of 'group think' may prevail which is not conducive to obtaining divergent views, the evaluator can exert less control over the process than is the case with one-to-one interviews and high quality recording and transcription are required if a reliable record is to be available to the evaluator. A detailed description of the use of focus groups and their strengths and weaknesses is provided by Morgan (1988).

Self-completion questionnaire

Self-completion questions are a relatively quick and straightforward way of receiving feedback as part of an evaluation. They are particularly suited to receiving feedback for formative purposes, for instance, from participants in a group activity. For detailed and thoughtful assessments of the overall worth of a project they are less powerful. It is important to remember that questionnaires are always time-consuming to design and require careful development to ensure that they collect useful and relevant information. An evaluator will also have to work hard to encourage a high and representative response rate.

Participant observation and journals

Participant observation is a technique used extensively by anthropologists. It aims to uncover, make accessible and reveal the meaning people use to make sense out of their daily lives (Jorgensen, 1989). It would be very rare that an evaluation budget would provide for an evaluator to spend the time necessary for effective participant observation. Key players within a project may be willing to become observers in a more systematic way than they might normally. For instance, journals kept by key staff on a community-based health promotion initiative can be an invaluable source of evaluation data as well as a useful tool for a reflective practitioner. Analysis of journal entries can provide a more accurate guide to the progress of the project than memories and assist in the reconstruction of the narrative of the project. Feelings and insights made at different points in a project may assist in explaining the directions taken by the project. The data from a journal or other means of recording observation are typically rich and detailed and assist an evaluator in bringing an initiative to life. The value of recording impressions over time was shown in a Ph.D. study of a participatory health promotion exercise amongst Australian blue-collar workers. The researcher made the following observation following one of her regular visits to a blast furnace at the steel works where she was conducting her study:

> It is fascinating it is taking up so much of their enthusiasm ... I left the furnace about four, went down and signed off with (the superintendent)

and came home feeling, yet again, amazed at the co-operation, enthusiasm, openness and I suppose effectiveness of these (last) two visits ...
One other thing (the superintendent) said to me: 'If you do want to take
photos here then that's OK.' Before I had been told it was inappropriate
to take photos. (This was) another indication of them feeling trust in my
not divulging and not breaching confidentiality.

(Ritchie, 1996, p. 153)

Written sources of data

There are many written sources of data that will be useful to an evaluator.
These include minutes of meetings, annual reports, newsletters and media
reports. These data can assist in constructing a narrative, checking the accu-
racy of other forms of data and indicate whether objectives have been achieved.
For instance, in the evaluation of a Healthy Cities project media coverage in
two areas were compared to determine whether the coverage of environmental and social health issues had increased more in the Healthy City community than in a comparison one (Baum and Cooke, 1992).

Validity of evaluation

It is crucial for an evaluator to be able to defend the validity of the data they
collect and use as the basis of their evaluation report. The use of a number of
different methods enables triangulation of the different data sources which
increase the validity of an evaluation. A further means of validation which is
important in community development is through the process of checking the
data with key participants in the particular initiative. This process is typically
used to reflect on and make changes to the way of working. It enables people
to play a role in the evaluation and will increase ownership of the evaluation
findings.

Validity is also increased through the process of critical thinking by all
participants in the evaluation. To be critical does not mean attacking the initiative
but, rather, reflecting on the meaning of the data collected for the evaluation
in a way that questions taken-for-granted-assumptions.

MAKING SENSE OF EVALUATION DATA

Writing the final evaluation report is generally the most challenging part of an
evaluation. It requires skills in critical analysis, political sensitivity and the
ability to make sense of divergent perspectives from different forms of data.
The evaluator will usually be seeking out themes and patterns that will assist
with understanding and interpretation, rather than trying to measure
precisely.

A useful report will generally provide a description of the initiative's process and key outcomes. It should describe the project's achievements and failings (most initiatives will have a mix of both) and then provide an overall assessment of the worth of the initiative.

Five criteria by which to judge participatory development projects put by Oakley (1991, pp. 17–18) will, in many circumstances, provide a useful framework by which to make this summative assessment of a community-based health promotion initiative. These five criteria are:

Efficiency

Participation can increase efficiency because people are more likely to be interested in benefits of initiatives that they have helped define and develop. If local people are involved in projects it reduces the amount of time needed by paid professional staff, and so becomes a cost-effective option. Oakley adds a caution here, however, as he points out that community development can become an excuse for shifting the costs of services and development on to already resource deprived and poor communities. Evaluators can consider the extent to which the initiative has been efficient in these terms. Often the achievements of these projects stand out as extremely good value for money because they rely on such a small input.

Effectiveness

Community development can make initiatives more effective because the process allows people to have a voice in determining objectives, supporting project administration and making their local knowledge, skills and resources available. Health promotion that is imposed on people is rarely effective. An evaluation can document the extent to which this has been the case and show, through the use of examples, how participation has increased the effectiveness of the project.

Self-reliance

This refers to the positive effect on people of participating in community development in health projects. The participation can help to break dependency (which has characterised much health and welfare work in the past) and so promote self-awareness and confidence which will help people to examine their problems and be positive about solutions. Community development also involves individual development and will increase people's sense of control over issues which affect their lives, help them to learn how to plan and implement and equip them for participation at regional and national levels. This helps create social capital which is a hallmark of a healthy community. The evaluator can assess the extent to which this self-reliance has been encouraged and people enabled to acquire skills and confidence that they did not have before the project started.

Coverage

In the past health promotion has tended to be more successful in reaching those who are already relatively healthy. Community development offers a way of working with people who are the least healthy. So the evaluator should assess the success of the initiative in involving people who are more often excluded, document how successfully they were included and if there was successful inclusion what factors enabled this to happen. The evaluator would also note the ways in which the initiative hadn't achieved a broad coverage and why that was the case.

Sustainability

Experience from numerous development projects indicate that those that are externally motivated frequently fail to be sustained once the initial level of support is reduced or withdrawn. In situations where local people are the main dynamic the chances of sustainability are increased. Consequently a crucial issue for the evaluator is the sustainability of the initiative and the mechanisms that have been put into place to ensure that this happens. If the initiative is not sustainable the evaluation should suggest why this is the case and what may have ensured sustainablility.

This framework provides scope for the evaluator to make an overall assessment of the worth of the project and to do this within a framework which is likely to provide information useful to each of the key players in a community-based health promotion initiative.

Giving feedback is an important aspect of evaluation research. The ways in which this is done will play a significant part in determining the extent to which the evaluation data is used. It is helpful if methods for doing this can be negotiated in advance. If the feedback happens in such a way that those receiving it reject it then no action on the basis of the findings is likely. Ideally in an evaluation process there should be enough interaction to ensure that the key findings come as no surprise to any of the main parties involved. Possibly the sign of a good evaluation is when people comment 'I could have told you that.' While that is not very rewarding for the evaluator it is one indicator that they have conducted their evaluation effectively. Evaluations which are based on a participatory method will automatically feed back evaluation findings into those directly involved but they will still have to grapple with the issue of making their evaluation findings meaningful and acceptable to funders and others who are likely not to have been centrally involved in the participatory process.

CONCLUSION

Community-based health promotion has increased in popularity as a strategy in recent years. As methodologies drawn from traditional biomedical science are rarely appropriate, the key challenge for the evaluators of these initiatives is to understand their dynamics and the social processes at their heart. It is, therefore, crucial that an evaluator understand the political and organisational setting of the initiatives and use a mix of (usually) qualitative and quantitative methods to gain a firm grasp on the workings of the initiative. By doing this, evaluation has the potential to become a development tool for the project participants and to contribute to emerging knowledge about the ways in which this exciting style of health promotion can be best implemented to promote health.

Note

Thanks very much to Charlie Murray, Gwyn Jolley and Paul Laris for helpful comments on an earlier draft of this chapter.

References

Allison, K. R. and I. Rootman (1996). Scientific research and community participation in health promotion research: are they compatible? *Health Promotion International* 11 (4): 333–340.

Baum, F. (1988). Community based research for the new public health. *Health Promotion* 3 (3): 259–268.

Baum, F. (1992). Moving targets: evaluation of community development. *Health Promotion Journal of Australia* 2 (2): 10–15.

Baum, F. (1995). *Health for All: The South Australian Experience*. Kent Town, South Australia, Wakefield Press.

Baum, F. (1996). Research to support health promotion based on community development approaches, in D. Colquhoun and A. Kellehear (eds) *Health Research in Practice*. London. Chapman and Hall: 184–202.

Baum, F. and R. Cook (1992). Healthy Cities Australia: evaluation of the pilot project in Noarlunga, South Australia. *Health Promotion International* 7 (3): 181–193.

Baum, F., D. Fry and I. Lennie (1992). *Community Health Policy and Practice in Australia*. Sydney, Pluto Press in conjunction with Australian Community Health Association.

Baum, F., C. Sanderson and G. Jolley (1997). Evaluation of the South Australian Health and Social Welfare Council Program. *Health Promotion International*. 12 (2): 125–134.

Boutilier, M., R. Mason and I. Rootman, (1997). Community action and reflective practice in health promotion research. *Health Promotion International* 12 (1): 69–78.

Brown, J., A. Collins and P. Duguid (1989). Situated cognition and the culture of learning. *Educational Researcher* 18, 1: 32–42.

Colin, T. and A. Garrow (1996). *Thinking, Listening, Looking, Understanding and Acting as You Go Along*. Alice Springs, Council of Remote Area Nurses of Australia Inc.

Community Development in Health (1988). *Community Development in Health: Resource Collection*. Melbourne, Community Development in Health.

Dixon, J. (1989). The limits and potential of community development for personal and social change. *Community Health Studies* 13 (1): 82–92.

Dwyer, J. (1989). The politics of participation. *Community Health Studies* 13 (1): 59–65.

Farquhar, J. W. *et al.* (1984). The Stanford Five Cities project: an overview. In J.D. Matarazzo *et al. Behavioural Health: A Handbook of Health Enhancement and Disease Prevention.* New York, John Wiley.

Feuerstein, M.-T. (1986). *Partners in Evaluation: Evaluating Development and Community Programmes with Participants.* London, Macmillan.

Freire, P. (1972). *Pedagogy of the Oppressed.* Harmondsworth, Penguin.

Fry, D. (1989). *Is There a Distinctive Community Health Approach to Health Promotion?* Health Promotion – the Community Health Approach, Melbourne, Australian Community Health Association.

Furler, E. (1979). Against Hegemony in Health Care Service Evaluation. *Community Health Studies* 3, 1: 32–341.

Hunt, Sonja (1987). Evaluating a community development project: issues of acceptability, *British Journal of Social Work* 17, 661–667.

Ife, J. (1995). *Community Development. Creating Community Alternatives – Vision, Analysis and Practice.* Melbourne, Longman.

Jackson, T., S. Mitchell *et al.* (1989). The community development continuum. *Community Health Studies* 13 (1): 66–73.

Jorgensen, D. I. (1989). *Participant Observation.* Newbury Park, California, Sage.

Kemmis, S. and R. McTaggart (1988). *The Action Research Planner.* Melbourne, Deakin University.

Kennedy, A. (1995) Measuring health for all – a feasibility study in a Glasgow community in N. Bruce, J. Springett, J. Hotchkiss and A. Scott-Samuel (eds) *Research and Change in Urban Community Health.* Aldershot, Avebury.

de Koning, K. and M. Martin (eds) (1996). *Participatory Research in Health: Issues and Experiences.* London, Zed Books.

Labonte, R. (1992). Heart health inequalities in Canada: models, theory and planning. *Health Promotion International* 7 (2): 119–127.

Labonte, R. and J. Feather (1996). *Handbook on Using Stories in Health Promotion Practice.* Prairie Region Health Promotion Research Centre, Canada, completed under contract with Health Canada.

Legge, D., G. Wilson *et al.* (1996). *Best Practice in Primary Health Care.* Melbourne, Centre for Development and Innovation in Health and Commonwealth Department of Health and Family Services.

Lincoln, Y. S. (1992). Sympathetic connections between qualitative connections and health research. *Qualitative Health Research* 2: 375–391.

Marsden, D. and P. Oakley (1991). Future issues and perspectives in the evaluation of social development. *Community Development Journal* 26, 4: 315–328.

Mayo, M. and G. Craig (1995). Community participation and empowerment: the human face of structural adjustment or tools for democratic transformation? In G. Craig and M. Mayo *Community Empowerment: A reader in Participation and Development.* London, Zed Books: 1–11.

McWalters, N., C. Hurwood *et al.* (1989). Step by step on a piece of string: an illustration of community work as a social health strategy. *Community Health Studies* 13 (1): 23–33.

Minichiello, V., R. Aroni, E. Timewell and A. Loris (1990). *In-depth Interviewing.* Melbourne, Longman Cheshire.

Morgan, D. L. (1988). *Focus Groups as Qualitative Research.* Portland, Sage.

Nutbeam, D. *et al.* (1993). Maintaining evaluation designs in long-term community-based health promotion programs: the Heartbeat Wales experience. *Epidemiology and Community Health*, 47, 127–133.

Oakley, P. (1991) *Projects with People.* Geneva, ILO.

Parlett, M. (1981). Illuminative evaluation. In P. Reason and J. Rowan *Human Inquiry.* Chichester, John Wiley & Sons: 219–226.

Petersen, A. and D. Lupton (1996). *The New Public Health: Health and Self in the Age of Risk*. St Leonards NSW, Allen & Unwin.

Puska, P., A. Nissinen *et al*. (1985). The community-based strategy to prevent coronary heart disease; conclusions from the ten years of the North Karelia project. *Annual Review of Public Health* 6: 147–193.

Raeburn, J. (1992). Health promotion research with heart; keeping a people perspective. *Canadian Journal of Public Health* 83 (Suppl.): S20–S24.

Ritchie, Jan (1996). A blast furnace is a blast furnace, y'know: promoting health in an industrial setting. Unpublished Ph.D. thesis, School of Medical Education, University of New South Wales.

Sanderson, C. and K. Alexander (1995). Community health services planning. In F. Baum *Health for all: the South Australian experience*. Adelaide, Wakefield Press: 161–171.

Sheills, A. and P. Hawe (1996). Health promotion, community development and the tyranny of individualism. *Health Economics*, 5, 141–147.

South Australian Community Health Research Unit (1997). *Evaluation of the South Australian Primary Health Care Initiatives and Advancement Program, 1994–5*. Adelaide, SACHRU.

Spradley, J. P. (1979). *The Ethnographic Interview*. New York. Holt, Rinehart & Winston.

Tesoriero, F. (1995). Community development and health promotion. In F. Baum *Health for All: the South Australian Experience*. Adelaide, Wakefield Press: 268–280.

Wadsworth, Y. (1984). *Do It Yourself Social Research*. Melbourne, Victorian Council of Social Services.

Wadsworth, Y. (1991). *Everyday Evaluation on the Run*. Melbourne, Action Research Issues Association (Inc.).

Wass, A. (1994). *Promoting Health: The Primary Health Care Approach*. Sydney, Harcourt Brace and Co.

Winkelstein, W. and M. Marmot (1981). Primary prevention of ischaemic heart disease: evaluation of community interventions. *Annual Review of Public Health* 2: 253–276.

World Health Organization (1986). The Ottawa Charter for Health Promotion. *Health Promotion* 1 (4): i–v.

Part II

Methods for assessing quality

Chapter 5

A quality assurance instrument for practitioners

An example from Sweden

Bo J.A. Haglund, Bjarne Jansson, Bosse Pettersson and Per Tillgren

Quality assurance can, on the one hand, be oriented towards a search for excellence; on the other, focus on improving performance in general health promotion work. Health promotion encompasses a philosophy, democratic values, policy structures and individual behaviours, and also a variety of methods. Since health promotion activities are rarely repeated, but are normally unique in terms of place, time and people, they have more in common with dynamic process development than regular service provision. This means that quality in health promotion must be assured even when activities are being designed and planned, so that the creation of optimal conditions for successful outcomes is facilitated. The importance of sharing experiences from local projects in a standardised and systematic way was stressed at the Third International Conference on Health Promotion in Sundsvall, Sweden, in 1991. A specific questionnaire, based on the Supportive Environments Action Model (SESAME), which is a stepwise action model with a focus on quality aspects, was used to build a database comprising more than 1,000 local health promotion projects worldwide. The 20-item questionnaire covered project planning, processes and outcomes. It has since been tested and revised, and now has six dimensions covering different aspects of quality: organisational quality; strategic quality; quality in approaching inequalities; quality of methods; and quality of monitoring and outcome measurement and quality improvement. Its use in local health promotion projects has demonstrated the instrument. So far, it has been employed in several health promotion settings, including healthy school development. The instrument has also been used (for training purposes) in health promotion courses at Masters level (MPH) and for experienced practitioners (in-service training) at the Karolinska Institute in Sweden.

INTRODUCTION

The scope of health promotion is broad. Philosophically, it deals with a positive concept of health, the fundamental principle of equal access to health opportunities, and also gender sensitivity. At one end, it encompasses multi-sectoral collaboration, at the other, the development of health-communication messages. Means range from public policy to furthering individual skills for living a healthy life. All this requires that any particular quality-assurance intervention in health promotion has to be developed on its own merits, taking the breadth of the area into account.

At present, there are a number of groups around the world discussing quality assurance issues in health promotion practice (Macdonald 1996a, 1996b, 1997). These discussions have already led to the production of practical manuals (Evans *et al.*, 1997; Van Driel and Keijsers, 1997). Ovretveit (1996) argues that two 'quality paradigms' are currently being debated: the External Standard Inspection (ESI) approach, and the Total Quality Management (TQM) model, in the hands of the executing organisation. A key question is which, if either, of these two 'paradigms' is most appropriate for assessing and improving the quality of any particular health promotion programme (Kahan, 1996).

The initial focus points of departure for our presentation concerns two significant problem-characteristics connected with quality improvement in the arena of health promotion. First, health promotion, when a multi-sectoral approach is adopted, includes co-operation between several different organisations. Each organisation has its own goals and practices. Several of the established QA instruments (ISO 14 000 and TQM) are designed for analysing a single company or organisation, not co-operation between several of them. The currently available instruments encompass leadership, information, strategic planning, staff training, working processes, results, and customer satisfaction. However, such comprehensive instruments (based, as they are on structure–process–outcome) are difficult to handle in minor, clearly delimited projects – largely due to low compliance. This applies especially during (rare) moments of political interest and economic investment in health. Yet, it is a common situation.

Second, the prerequisites for (local) general health promotion work at different national levels differ between communities and change over time. Many HP projects and activities are built on some previous experiences – more or less systematically recorded and considered – and designs are seldom repeated. Accordingly, the impact of health promotion activities in practice is unclear and unpredictable, and needs to be subject to continuous review. A project-oriented instrument should therefore have a design which enables a critical attitude to be adopted towards planning and analysing such activities.

Ideally, a QA instrument should provide an opportunity to scrutinise single parts of a project without losing an overall organisational perspective. When applying an extensive instrument developed for and by QA experts there is a significant risk of low compliance if projects involve people with limited training and experience. The aim of this chapter is to present an instrument which might be used in practice without specific training in quality-assurance management. The instrument can be handled after just two days training: one day to provide a theoretical basis for the approach, and instructions on how to use the manual; one further day of follow-up, with health planners testing the instrument in their own setting and practice.

THE QUALITY CONCEPT WITHIN A HEALTH PROMOTION CONTEXT

In the heading for this chapter the term Quality Assurance has been purposely chosen. A number of terms in the 'quality field' are used and related, such as:

- Quality Standards (QS), understood as what level of quality ambition is expected to be met (e.g. functional, good, excellent) and further expressed as criteria and indicators.
- Quality Management (QM) and Total Quality Management (TQM), understood as how to manage the (whole) process, and how to secure that the level of agreed quality is met – and by evaluation identify potentials for quality improvement as well as more efficient implementation procedures.
- Quality Assessment (QAs), understood as by which means monitoring and evaluation is carried out, as well as the results.
- Quality Control (QC), understood both as how the control is monitored continuously as well as the control of the final outcome, related to agreed QS.
- Quality Assurance (QA), understood as the methodology to secure quality in health promotion, mainly by focusing on the planning phase of activities and projects.
- Quality Improvement (QI), understood as how to gain from the evaluation analysis, in order to improve the planning of subsequent activities.

In most of the common health promotion activities run by practitioners, these concepts can be illustrated and related in the following model (Figure 5.1). In the ideal case there is a team responsible for the different phases of a health promotion activity, with special competence in different parts like planning, implementation, monitoring and evaluation and quality management. If not, in favourable circumstances, external competence is both available and affordable. However, in practice it may well be that the single health planner has to be responsible for carrying out the whole process. In such cases a more realistic and feasible approach is to develop a QA instrument, which to a reasonable extent also embraces other dimensions of quality management. The critical prerequisites to assure the quality of a health promotion activity are:

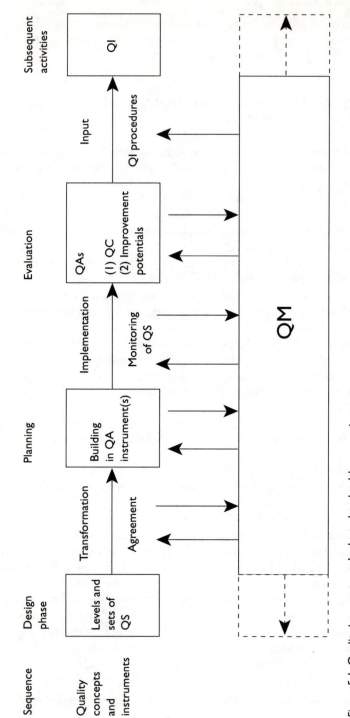

Figure 5.1 Quality 'concept map' adapted to health promotion

1   to build in QA instruments as a core element in the planning process –
    any later attempt will fail by definition,
2   to agree upon the quality standard (in terms of level of ambition),
    what indicators and criteria to be used in the monitoring and evaluation
    procedures, and
3   to consider the nature and specific features of health promotion,
    compared with health services, consumer products etc., when one of the
    main characteristics is the dynamic process orientation. Thus, the ability
    to respond flexibly becomes an important quality criterion.

QUALITY MODELS IN OTHER DISCIPLINES

As an introduction, we address the framework of QA models and the concepts which, in general, are agreed to be relevant in the field of health promotion and public health. It is argued that each of the concepts referred to below
have obvious shortcomings when applied to health promotion as we have
described it. Nevertheless, they make major contributions, both systematic
and particular, and demonstrate indirectly why quality assurance in health
promotion has a rationale of its own.

Models for health-care systems

Donobedian's model for health care has been used as a foundation for several instruments. The model emphasises the importance of factors which
directly and indirectly influence the health result (outcome): 'Care must be
taken to hold all significant factors other than medical care constant if valid
conclusions are to be drawn.' Further, the importance of 'using measures of
process' is stressed, on the grounds that these are 'more readily available'
than 'measures of outcome'. This requires, however, that 'the process measures chosen have a valid and stable relationship with outcome measures and
that they can therefore be used as appropriate proxy for outcomes'
(Donobedian, 1966).

Sheps (1955) has stressed the importance of defining the purposes of quality
assessment. She emphasised that the methods and measures selected must be
appropriate to the objectives of the assessment. If the objective is an application
for accreditation, the instrument must distinguish between 'good enough' and
'not good enough' (quality assessment of a critical borderline). But, if the
purpose is to stimulate quality improvements, it is not enough to distinguish
between poor and excellent. Then, the instrument must also contribute to the
identification of specific areas of improvement, i.e. things about which something
must be done (quality improvement).

In the course of the development of the 'medical audit', a distinction was
made between the use of 'explicit' criteria (agreed in advance by a group of

interested persons, possibly including those whose work is to be audited) and 'implicit' criteria (subjective judgements according to evidence available at the time). Further criteria, suggested by Sanazaro (1974), hinge on the distinction between 'optimal care' and 'essential care'. The former comprises elements of care which may be necessary to guarantee good care, but a low rating on any one of them does not necessarily indicate poor care under particular circumstances. The latter comprises those elements which are regarded as essential to proper care in all circumstances. However, one analysis of health-care purchasing shows that few purchasers, and also few researchers or policy-makers, consider quality to be significant in the purchasing arena (Ovretveit, 1995). Among other things this point is in the gap between professional and political ambitions on the one hand, and shortcomings in the implementation on the other.

Implicitly, the models are founded on a 'what's best for others' approach; i.e. the attitude is paternalistic. Paternalism in this context refers to an activity developed and practised with the intention of benefiting a recipient, but without his or her informed consent (Kikki, 1997).

QA of products in health promotion and disease prevention

Health promotion and disease prevention are concerned with both prod-ucts and services. For example, medical drug therapies involves pharmaceu-ticals; safety promotion involves the manufacturing of products such as fire alarms, safety seats for children in cars, and life-jackets; promotion of sexu-ality and family planning involves contraceptives; and diet promotion in-volves the preparation of low-fat/high-fibre foods, etc. Responsibility for product quality rests on the manufacturer. Quality assurance for health pro-motion products is largely the same as for other consumer goods, but with one important addition. Since these products are concerned with life or death – either instantly or in the long run – demands are exceptionally high. In most countries, the objects involved are subject to special control. In some cases the quality (specified criteria met) may be controlled by govern-mental authorities, and in other cases by acknowledged neutral private bod-ies. Most health promoters are not too much concerned with these aspects, since neither do they fall into their field of competence nor are they a major problem in general. (There are, of course, exceptions such as 'healthy' ciga-rettes, alcopops, and food products labelled and marketed under specifica-tions they do not meet.) Probably the most important roles health promoters can play in improving product quality are to formulate demands which can improve the function of products, to make 'good' products more widely used, and to campaign so that such products are economically available to those most in need.

Health promotion applied to service production quality criteria

Information and persuasion in health education can be looked upon as service production. Accordingly, there is a need at the outset to define the concept of 'service'. From the literature, several features of the concept of service can be distinguished (Grönroos, 1992). Services are regarded as intangible assets, i.e. they cannot be stored (perishability), they are difficult to standardise (heterogeneity), and they can be seen as a chain of activities (intangibility). Production and consumption take place simultaneously (inseparability). The most distinct feature of the concept lies in the association between service and ' human relations' (Edvardsson and Gummesson, 1988; Gummesson, 1991). A wide variety of different kinds of services are offered by both the public and private sectors. Measurement of service quality presupposes a good understanding of the content of any particular service, facilitating identification of what is essential to it and what is possible to measure it (Gummesson, 1993). These aspects are important to bear in mind when planning health promotion activities.

Health promotion and 'customer quality' service

Quality is about both obvious, measurable characteristics and accompanying and concealed factors. Customers' perceptions of level of quality are central (Juran, 1992). In principle, it should not be more difficult to measure the quality of services than that of products. One problem, however, is lack of experience of systematic QA of service production (Gummesson, 1993). Service quality can be divided into four main parts. Construction quality (A) comprises a specification of service content and practicability. Production quality (B) is concerned with how well a producer delivers various services. In these two respects, it is essential to do the right things from the beginning. A majority (90 per cent) of faults in industry can be assigned to the construction phase (Deming, 1986), and the same conclusion has been drawn for the service sector (Crosby, 1979). Good planning is therefore crucial, especially under unstable circumstances. Relation quality (C) is about adequate treatment of the customer. Technical quality (D) concerns the future usefulness of the service. Both these latter aspects are of relevance in health promotion work.

There are a number of related quality concepts. Quality control tries to identify the gap between customers' expectations and producers' understanding of these expectations (Zeithaml *et al.*, 1990). For example, the content of a health education programme may not in practice fulfil its audience's expectations of the programme. The primary purpose of quality measurement is to initiate improvement, and its methods can be employed to facilitate achievement of the goals of QA. However, this is seldom the experience in practice. Benchmarking, which is concerned with how to increase capacity to promote competition, is a common tool in industry (Camp, 1989). Comparing outcomes between your own organisation and others is intended to effect better self-analytic capability and to disseminate standards of excellence. A model for comparing processes in industry has been developed by Watson (1992). There are clear similarities between benchmarking and conducting research. The relevance for health promotion is obvious in comparing larger and theory-based programmes with well developed structures and implementation strategies.

A number of quality dimensions for services have also been presented (Zeithaml *et al.*, 1990). These are reliability, sensitiveness, competence, availability, performance, communication, trustworthiness, safety and correction. All can be used in health promotion. Methods of surveillance include observation, interviews, questionnaires, focus-group interviews, problem-detection studies, and case studies.

However, a major dilemma remains. The customer of health promotion is not of one kind only – it comprises individuals, groups, but also communities and when it comes to 'purchasing' it includes politicians and decision-makers.

The objectives of health promotion are relatively simple to formulate. Health promotion is about increasing exposures that contribute to health and quality of life. However, achieving goals is dependent on co-operation between several different interests in society, and it is not always possible to make these converge. This should mainly be considered during the planning process.

THE QUALITY CONTEXT IN HEALTH PROMOTION

Quality aspects of health promotion are receiving increasing attention in Sweden. One major reason for this is competition for scarce resources. In more and more institutions, it is necessary to claim and demonstrate good quality standards to get proposals accepted. A further important reason is the professionalisation of health promotion practitioners – due to training and other capacity-enhancing measures. As a result, there is an increased use of theory-based models for different interventions and in large-scale projects.

Quality assurance might be encapsulated in the saying: 'Doing things right is not enough if the right things are not done correctly.' Putting it more precisely, the sentence should read something like: 'Doing the right things correctly means having an explicit level of expectations in terms of standard criteria, combined with fair resources and other necessary prerequisites.' This provides an understanding of the essence of the concept of quality when applied to health promotion and other non-repetitive services.

The context in which quality standards are applied can be viewed from at least three angles (Pettersson and Omberg, 1997):

1   QA is, at least to a certain degree, a manageable tool for securing and facilitating a certain standard in advance by setting criteria in order to forecast a variable outcome ranging from acceptable to excellent, in the light of specific difficulties for different undertakings, ambitions and given

resources (and other) inputs. This might be referred to as the 'Volkswagen–Rolls-Royce approach'.

2 QA is a scientifically – and also politically – attractive method for offering a guarantee that certain predictable mistakes will not be made. This might be referred to as the 'warranty approach.'

3 QA can essentially be regarded as part of a four-cornered and inter-linked set of relations between specific quality criteria and standards (1), project management, planning and competence of the organisation (2), training (3), and evaluation (4).

In many cases, there seems to be confusion both about different quality definitions and, for example, about whether quality assurance is the same as quality evaluation. In the long run, the relation between the two may be the opposite to what one might expect. The idea of quality assurance is to secure planning tools and 'production' processes up to a limit where specific standard criteria are met. In the ideal case, it should be possible to forecast to a 99.9 per cent degree of certainty that an outcome will meet initially defined expectations. Quality assurance, by means of quality criteria and specific standards, provides a shortcut to expected and desired outcome(s). But this is the case only for routine-based and repetitive services, which arise only rarely in the arena of health promotion.

What aspects of quality assurance are specific to health promotion?

A fundamental issue in discussing quality assurance in relation to health promotion is whether QA theories and models have any specific features when applied in the field. At least three different features can be identified.

One, in relation to the production of both products and services, is that quality standards are generally developed for and applied to routine and repetitive procedures. We can find such situations in health promotion, e.g. standardised programmes for school health education, but even there characteristics and circumstances differ from one school setting to another. Health promotion projects are generally unique, and never repeated in their original design. Any second attempt is, and is hopefully reported and reviewed as, a next step in quality improvement, and so on.

A second feature is that the targeted consumer/user/client of population-oriented health promotion lacks a clear 'voice'. Quality standards are – and should be – set by those who demand action, whether they be politicians or the high-level officials who act as purchasers or decision-makers in a traditional organisational model. Ultimately, it is these same persons who are presumed to represent the public. We have to admit that usually, although perhaps not always, the voice of the target group cannot be sufficiently heard.

A third feature is that 'professional' standards may attach to health promotion practitioners. Such standards hopefully exist, but will certainly vary between different categories of health promoters. The reason for this is that much of health promotion is value-driven, and there is no single agreed basic philosophy to provide a common foundation. Consequently, interpretation of quality will differ between health promoters according to the philosophies to which they adhere.

Table 5.1 is an attempt to catch and compare some of the characteristics when different determinants of QA is translated into health promotion and related to health services and consumer products. It is obvious that there is a need to further develop QA instruments, departing from the nature of health promotion.

Table 5.1 Ten examples: comparative interpretations of some items approaching QA for health promotion related to health services and consumer products

Item	Health services	Consumer products	Health promotion
1 Client	Individuals	Potential consumers	Individuals, groups, populations, public, environment, communities etc.
2 Product	Standards defined by profession	Standardised Defined by physics, applied usefulness	Open dynamic process Defined by environment and involved partners
3 Standards	Agreed, classified	Strictly defined	Variety of models
4 Valuebase	Biomedical science	Competitive commercial	Social, political
5 Skills	Nursing, caring, treatment	Manufacturing, entrepreneur	Generalistic, entrepreneur
6 Frequence	Repetitive	Continuous	One-by-one
7 Organisation	Monolithic, Professional hierarchy	Monolithic, Productivity focused	Pluralistic Inter/multi sectoral Facilitation
8 Management focus	Safety	Competition	Empowerment Equity in health
9 'Environment'	Standardised setting e.g. hospital	Mechanised setting e.g. factory	Altering settings e.g. schools, workplaces
10 Outcome	Successful treatment	Profit	Desired structural, environmental and behavioural changes

TOOLS AND MANUALS FOR QUALITY STANDARDS

The theories of quality assessment in disease prevention and health promotion tend to borrow their role models from medical care. Surprisingly or not! However, these models (quality circles and others), despite their visual simplicity, are too complicated to put into health promotion practice in most cases. They are also too narrow, in the sense that they apply more to strictly defined operations (e.g. surgery) than to processes where dynamics play a given and somewhat unpredictable role. Quality assurance in health promotion must account for these dynamics, both as a reality which takes experience to manage, and as offering an opportunity to apply creative solutions so as to effect outcome improvements.

In Sweden, at least four manuals (or other tools) have been developed, all of which take a practitioner's perspective:

1   *The Sundsvall Handbook* (Haglund *et al.*, 1993) was developed in conjunction with the Third International Conference on Health Promotion (1991), and contains the '20-item questionnaire' referred to above. Originally, the manual was designed as a model for reporting data on health promotion projects to various databases. When tested among health planners in the county of Västernorrland, however, it was noted that the model also functioned well as a planning tool with in-built critical quality items. It is now used in training and for regular reporting in different parts of Sweden. It will be discussed below and presented in detail in the appendix to this chapter.

2   A simple check list of a 'dozen quality components' has been presented by Pettersson (1992) for training purposes. The list covers a series of aspects: initial strategic intents and targets applied to the Donabedian concept (structure–process–outcome), strategic judgements and situation analysis, transparency in priority setting, feasibility and effectiveness, ethics, available competence, organisation and collaboration, theory-based methodology, and systematic performance (including monitoring, evaluation and drawing conclusions relevant to future undertakings). In addition, there are discussions of whether quality-improving innovations as such can be planned at all, and of the responsibility of decision-makers (and purchasers) to make future use of the productive and successful experiences gained from pilot projects.

3   *Succeeding with Health Promotion Projects: Quality Assurance* (Landstingsförbundet, 1996) is a manual published by the Federation of County Councils in Sweden. It builds more strictly on the Donabedian 1996 concept of 'structure–process–outcome', which is translated into specific cases, and then generalised into a questionnaire. The manual was developed by experienced MPH students. It has been officially

recognised, and some public-health units in Sweden have obtained funding support for health promotion projects conditional upon its use.

4   Based on its nation-wide surveillance remit with regard to the public-health undertakings of county councils, county administrative boards and municipalities, Sweden's National Board of Health and Welfare reported in 1994 on how the Swedish county councils were fulfilling their responsibilities. The main observation was that the councils did not regularly report, monitor or evaluate their activities concerned with disease prevention or health promotion. In order to promote and facilitate interest in quality improvement, the National Board published a booklet in 1995 called *Quality in Disease Prevention and Health Promotion* (in Swedish only). The booklet discusses the concept of quality, gives examples of terminology in use (thereby illustrating some of the current conceptual confusion), describes the various stages in quality assurance (illustrated by actual cases), presents development methods, and finally shows the applicability of different methods to disease prevention and health promotion.

Other instruments have been developed in Europe. One is the so-called PREFFI instrument, 'Prevention Effectiveness Instrument' produced in The Netherlands (Van Driel and Keijsers, 1997). The Dutch model has a specific focus on health education and individual behaviour.

   A UK project to develop a framework for quality assurance in health promotion practice emphasises six key functions of health promotion: strategic planning; programme management; monitoring and evaluation; education and training; resources and information; and advice and consultancy (Speller *et al.*, 1997; Speller *et al.* in this volume).

THE 20-ITEM QUESTIONNAIRE

One of the key themes of the Sundsvall conference concerned how to find innovative ways of sharing experiences on how to create healthy environments through systematised storytelling. Narratives on how to create supportive environments for health became a central element in the conference edition of *The Sundsvall Handbook, 'We Can Do It!'* (Haglund *et al.*, 1993), which represented the main outcome of the conference. This was later published by WHO as number 3 in the Public Health in Action series under the title *Creating Supportive Environments for Health: Stories from the Third International Conference on Health Promotion*, Sundsvall, Sweden (Haglund *et al.*, 1996). The importance of systematised storytelling has been highlighted by Kickbusch in her introductory chapter, 'Tell me a story' in the book, *Health Promotion in Canada* (Pedersen *et al.*, 1994). The author claims that stories open up opportunities for ownership and identification, and also provide the courage to effect change. This is especially so when the stories are about where people live, love, work, and play – in short, about everyday life (Kickbusch, 1994). The storytelling technique has been refined by means of practical tests in Sweden, the results of which are presented in the form of 'Twenty Key Items for Health Promotion Actions' – the questionnaire for systematisation of knowledge and experiences on creating 'Supportive Environments for Health' presented in the appendix to this chapter. Since 1994, Labonte and Feather have further developed what they call the 'Story-Dialogue Method' for knowledge development and evaluation, largely through the production of a theoretical framework for the use of systematised storytelling and practical experiment (Labonte and Feather, 1996). The methods used are based on Freire's reflections on raising critical consciousness through the basic principles of 'see', 'reflect', and 'act' (Freire, 1968). In the context of QA this methodology applies to how to improve quality by gaining from earlier experiences and observations.

Developing the 20-item questionnaire

The origin of the 20-item questionnaire lay in the need (1) to systematise the stories told to the Sundsvall conference in 1991 by participants and other committed health promoters around the world, and (2) to develop a structure for how to build databases in a standardised but yet simple manner so as to facilitate the sharing of experiences among HP practitioners.

When analysing the stories, it became apparent that certain features were given greater prominence than others when the storyteller explained why the action was successful. The initial ambition and idea was to use the analysed material to construct a database (which was achieved in Sundsvall on the basis of the stories told). The next step was to condense the data within a comprehensive structure, simple enough to be managed by standard PCs and shareware programmes.

At this time (1991–92), the QA concept was not well recognised among health promoters. The first version of the questionnaire was built on eight main items (with additional sub-items) and published in the Conference Edition of the Sundsvall Handbook (Haglund *et al.*, 1993). The questionnaire was tested during a five-day session of follow-up in-service training for health planners held in the county of Västernorrland. After testing and practising with the questionnaire, some of the health planners expressed the view that 'it was a shame they hadn't had and used these before'. 'Then,' in their view, 'a lot of misjudgements and mistakes could have been avoided.' From that time onwards, the development of the questionnaire shifted in focus from the reporting of experiences to considering key issues for quality improvement and thus securing a more successful outcome of health promotion activities. The form has been continuously refined and tested in practice and has been found to be useful in both to stimulate improved planning of action taken by health planners and to record it in a systematised way.

Since the questionnaire draws attention to equity questions the equality dimension is highlighted. The dimension of inequalities in health seems not to be well covered in other QA instruments. Whether it is used for sharing experiences or as a tool for quality assurance depends on the approach adopted. But, at the end of the day, these are two sides of the same coin, and the outcome is likely to be improvement of the quality in both cases.

Good planning: a QA prerequisite

Quality assurance can only be built in during the planning phase of an activity. In the case of the 20-item questionnaire reference is made to the 'Supportive Environments Action Model' (SESAME). Influenced by research traditions in the social work arena, the model has been modified to become more sequential and take the form of a spiral (Swedner, 1982). SESAME is an action-oriented model for dynamic planning aiming at stepwise action to create supportive environments for health. It illustrates a logical, universal sequence of actions which incorporates many fields of human activities (see Figure 5.2).

Many everyday as well as professional activities follow a natural, logical stepwise process, which we all recognise. Basically, the process consists of three stages: identifying a problem, reflecting on solutions, and acting to solve the problem.

SESAME is temporal; it is based on an orderly progression of logical steps in a time sequence. The reason why some steps, e.g. target-setting, strategy

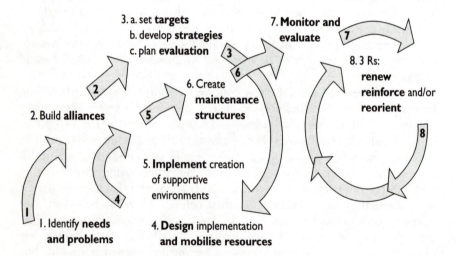

Figure 5.2 Supportive environments action model (SESAME)
Source: Haglund *et al.* (1993).

development, and evaluation planning (3a–c), have been combined into one item rather than remaining separate, is that integration make sense. Much health promotion is based on participation by involvement from communities and partners already, from the very first step. If, and when such aspects are considered as important qualities of an undertaking, they must also be enabled by the planning model.

Quality dimensions in the 20-item questionnaire

The instrument has six quality dimensions: (1) organisational structure; (2) strategic intents – by setting of objectives and targets, and defining primary and secondary target groups; (3) quality in focusing – or not – inequalities and gender sensitivity; (4) appropriateness and combination of methods; (5) quality of monitoring and outcome procedures, and (6) quality improvement (see Table 5.2). In this presentation, however, the SESAME model has been used to structure these dimensions:

- *Organisational quality* is concerned with the prerequisites of participating partners, joint funding, and maintenance. If collaborative partnership is lacking in an undertaking involving different actors, then one important quality aspect – multi-sectoral action – is missing right from the start of the project. Organising is a critical part for maintaining what is expected to follow after a time-limited project.
- *Strategic quality* means that rationale, strategic intents, and objectives and targets are clear and logically defined, understandable and agreed upon. Primary target groups where effects are expected (e.g. pupils) must be defined, as too must secondary target groups, i.e. the mediators (e.g. teachers).
- *Quality in reducing health inequities.* Equity in health is regarded by WHO, and also in many national public health steering documents, as the overall aim of different public-health strategies, including health promotion. Closely related is the issue of gender sensitivity. It is therefore important to clarify the extent to which equal opportunities for health and gender sensitivity are included in local plans and the actual implementation of health promotion work. Dimensions of ethnicity and the distribution of health between different geographical areas are also included here.
- *Quality of methods* concerns the relevance and appropriateness of methods planned for use in relation to objectives and targets.
- *Evaluation quality* with regard to monitoring and outcome measurement deals with relevance of methods employed and evaluation criteria.
- *Quality improvement* is focused by the storytelling method recognising main obstacles and explorative descriptions about how and what solutions were developed. This ends up in analytical conclusions for subsequent undertakings.

Table 5.2 Quality dimensions in the 20-item questionnaire

Quality dimension	Items (refer to no. of item in form)
A Organisational structure	Partners (coversheet), location and setting (4), initiative (9), funding (10), maintenance (18)
B Strategic considerations	Rationale for undertaking (5) goals and objectives (6), target groups (7)
C Equity focus	Approaching socio economic, gender, ethnic and geographical health differences (8).
D Relevant methodology	Strategies (11), means and methods for implementation (12)
E Quality control assessment	Monitoring (13), evaluation (14), impact (15)
F Improvement	Obstacles and solutions (17), (19), conclusions (20)

PERFORMANCE: SEARCH FOR EXCELLENCE AND GENERAL IMPACT

Two main directions of quality assurance can be identified. One aims at developing excellence, the other at affecting health promotion already in place. The search for excellence is the spearhead of development and is closely linked to research. It demands high competence, designated resources and is often limited to a defined specific area.

Improving the quality of health promotion – as well as health promoters – is a challenge in order to influence the vast majority of what can be done in the form of 'business as usual' or in some better way. Achieving a 10 per cent improvement in what is already in place should have a major impact on the effectiveness of health promotion. The 20-item questionnaire can be an instrument of this kind.

In sum, the continuous improvement of health promotion is of central importance. Sometimes, similar results can be achieved in several ways. The preventive impact of many programmes is unknown, and then ongoing critical analysis is required. Health promotion is very much dependent on participants' shifting interests, knowledge, time and motivation. Instruments should be easy to handle and cost-effective so as to avoid 'one-shot' experiences. In the long run, documented awareness of successful and unsuccessful strategies will be of great importance to those who practise and finance HP programmes. Instruments need therefore to be adapted to the fact that health promotion involves many professionals – both skilled and unskilled.

Since several of the instruments developed in Sweden and elsewhere rely on practice, the basic structure of their items are rather similar. This is clear, for example, if we compare the different efforts made in Sweden with the Dutch PREFFI-instrument (Van Driel and Keijsers, 1997; Keijsers and Saan in this volume). However, there is a difference in focus between the two. The PREFFI model has its focus on health education, individual behaviour change, and related theories, whereas the 20-item questionnaire focuses on structural and environmental change based on community organisational theory.

However, the most critical quality component is the health promoter her/himself. Improving the quality of health promotion with substantial impact should be based on three cornerstones: first, professional training of health promoters, second, development, recognition and implementation of user-friendly instruments for practitioners, and third, QA instruments which are constructed from the nature and reality of health promotion.

References

Camp, R. (1989). Bench marking. The search for industry best practices that lead to superior performance. *Quality Progress* 22, January, 61–68, February 70–75, March 76–82, April 62–69.

Crosby P. (1979). *Quality is Free.* New York: McGraw-Hill.

Deming, W.E. (1986). *Out of the Crisis.* Cambridge, MA: MIT.

Donobedian, A. (1966). Evaluating the quality of medical care. *Milbank Memorial Fund Quarterly* 44, Supplement, 166–203.

Edvardsson, B. and Gummesson E. (1988). Management i tjänstesamhället – på väg mot en ny företagsekonomi, in Edvardsson, B. and Gummesson, E. (eds) *Management i tjänstesamhället.* Malmö: Liber (in Swedish).

Evans, D., Speller, V. and Head, M.J. (1997). Developing quality assurance standards for health promotion practice in the UK. *Health Promotion International* 12: 215–224.

Freire, P. (1968). *Pedagogy of the Oppressed.* New York: Seabury Press.

Grönroos, C. (1992). *Strategic Management.* Göteborg: ISL Förlag.

Gummesson, E. (1991). Kvalitetsstyrning i tjänste- och serviceverksamheter. *Forskningsrapport* 91: 4. Karlstad: CTF (in Swedish).

Gummesson, E. (1993). *Att förstÆ kundens upplevda kvalitet. Vad kan offentlig sektor lära av näringslivet?* Stockholm: Stockholms universitet. Företagsekonomiska institutionen (in Swedish).

Haglund, B.J.A., Pettersson, B., Finer, D. and Tillgren, P (1993). *The Sundsvall Handbook, 'We Can Do It!'* From the Third International Conference on Health Promotion, Sundsvall, Sweden, 9–15 June 1991. Sundbyberg: Karolinska Institutet, Department of Public Health Sciences, Division of Social Medicine.

Haglund, B.J.A., Pettersson, B., Finer D. and Tillgren, P. (1996). *Creating Supportive Environments for Health. Stories from the Third International Conference on Health Promotion, Sundsvall, Sweden.* No. 3 in Public Health Action series. Geneva: World Health Organization.

Juran, J.M. (1992). *Juran on Quality by Design.* New York: The Free Press.

Kahan, B. Memo (1996). *Continuous Quality Improvement and Health Promotion.* Toronto: University of Toronto, Department of Health Promotion.

Kickbusch, I. (1994). Tell me a story. In Pederson, A. O'Neill, M. and Rootman, I. (eds), *Health Promotion in Canada. Provincial, National and International Perspectives.* Toronto: W.B. Saunders Canada, 8–17.

Kikki, N. (1997). Informative paternalism: studies in the ethics of promoting and predicting health Ph.D. thesis. Tema Institute, Dept of Health and Society, Linköping University, Sweden.

Labonte, R. and Feather, J. (1996). *Handbook on Using Stories in Health Promotion Practice.* Ottawa: Health Canada.

Landstingsförbundet (1996). *Succeeding with Health Promotion Projects – Quality Assurance,*

Landstingsförbundet, Stockholm, Sweden. First published as: Ader, M., Berensson, K., Carlsson, P., Granath, M., Olsson-Enhorn, G. and Urwitz V. (1992) Kvalitetsindikatorer på befolkningsnivå. Skövde: Landstingets hälsovård rapport nr 26 (available in English).

Macdonald, G. (1996a) *Presentation of Existing Standards for Evaluation and Quality Assessment of Health Promotion Intervention in the 15 EU Member States. Final Report.* Woerden, Netherlands: International Union for Health Promotion and Education and Netherlands Institute for Health Promotion and Disease Prevention.

Macdonald, G.(1996b) *Presentation of Existing Standards for Evaluation and Quality Assessment of Health Promotion Intervention in the 15 EU Member States. Country Reports.* Woerden, Netherlands: International Union for Health Promotion and Education and Netherlands Institute for Health Promotion and Disease Prevention.

Macdonald, G.(1997) Quality indicators and health promotion effectiveness. *Promotion and Education* 4 (2): 5–8.

Ovretveit, J. (1995). *Purchasing for Health.* Buckingham: Open University Press.

Ovretveit, J. (1996). Quality in health promotion. *Health Promotion International* 1: 55–62.

Pedersen, A., O'Neill, M. and Rootman, I. (eds) (1994) *Health Promotion in Canada: Provincial, National and International Perspectives.* Toronto. W.B. Saunders, Canada.

Pettersson, B. (1992). *Ett dussin kvalitetskomponenter i hälsofrämjande arbete.* Working paper. Stockholm: Karolinska Institute, Department of Public Health Sciences, Division of Social Medicine – Master Course in Health Promotion (in Swedish).

Pettersson, B. and Omberg, L. (1997) *Observations on Development and Trends in H.P. Quality Issues in Sweden.* Sundbyberg: Department of Public Health Sciences, WHO Collaborating Centre on Supportive Environments for Health at the Karolinska Institute.

Sanazaro, P.J. (1974). Medical audit: experience in the USA. *British Medical Journal* 1: 271–274.

Sheps, M. (1955). Approaches to the quality of hospital care. *Public Health Reports,* 70: 877–886.

Speller, V., Evans, D. and Head, M. J. (1997) Developing quality assurance standards for health promotion practice in the UK. *Health Promotion International* 12 (3): 215–224.

Swedner, H. (1982). *Human Welfare and Action Research in Urban Settings.* Stockholm: Liber förlag.

Van Driel, W.G. and Keijsers, J.F.E.M. (1997). An instrument for reviewing the effectiveness of health education and health promotion. *Patient Education and Counselling* 30: 7–17.

Watson, G.H. (1992). *The Benchmarking Workbook.* Cambridge Massachusetts: Productivity Press.

Zeithaml, V.A., Parasuraman, A. and Berry, L.L. (1990). *Delivering Quality Service.* New York: The Free Press.

APPENDIX I

Learning from experiences: share your experiences

(From Haglund *et al.*, 1996.)

A Title of project/experience/activity

–Write here–

( ) Separate project
( ) The project is part of a larger programme/activity, namely …
Planned project ( )   Project in progress ( )   Completed project ( )

B The information herein is provided by:

Name (title):
Organisation/workplace:
Address (PO box no.):
Postal or zip code: City:
Tel. (incl. country and area code):
Country:
Fax (incl. country and area code):
E-mail address:

C Project leader (if different from above)

Name (title):
Organisation/workplace:
Address (PO box no.):
Postal or zip code: City:
Tel. (incl. country and area code):
Country:
Fax (incl. country and area code):
E-mail address:

D Contact person (if different from either of the above)

Name (title):
Organisation/workplace:
Address (PO Box no.):
Postal or zip code: City:
Tel. (incl. country and area code):
Country:
Fax (incl. country and area code):
E-mail address:

E Collaborative partner(s)

(Note: If there are several partners, continue overleaf or on separate piece of paper)
Name (title):
Organisation/workplace:
Address (PO box no.):
Postal or zip code: City:
Tel. (incl. country and area code):
Country:
Fax (incl. country and area code):
E-mail address:

Twenty items about projects on creating supportive environments for health

I Abstract

Briefly (maximum fifteen lines) describe the project. (Cover key information on questions 2 to 20, i.e. aim/objective, how the project was carried out (method of implementation), where and by whom; results and experiences; conclusion for the future, expected if ongoing)
[*Write here*]

2 Start (project started, year, month):

[*Write here*]

3 End (scheduled time of completion, year, month):

[*Write here*]

4 Locality and setting(s)

Where, i.e. county, municipality or part thereof and in which setting(s)/ arena(s), school(s), workplace(s), neighbourhood area, etc., was the project carried out?
[*Write here*]

5 Aim(s)

Main purpose (problems/needs) of the project?
[*Write here*]

6 Goals and objectives

What goal(s) and objectives did the project have in terms of its approach, and in terms of its effects?

[*Write here*]

7 Target group

Which group(s) were targeted by the project?

(a) Directly approached (e.g. agents, teachers):

   [*Write here*]

(b) Indirectly approached (e.g. students via teachers or agents):

   [*Write here*]

8 Equity focus

(a) Was the project explicitly directed towards increasing equity in health?

   Yes ( )   No ( )

(b) If yes, was it in terms of:

   groups (social, ethnic)   Yes ( )   No ( )

   geographical areas   Yes ( )   No ( )

   gender (men and women)   Yes ( )   No ( )

   other   Yes ( )   No ( )

If yes, please comment:

[*Write here*]

9 Initiative

Who/which organisations initiated the project/activity?

[*Write here*]

10 *Funding*

(a) What basic financing was available for the project? From where? (name several sources if funding was supplied by other than the responsible main project organisation)

[*Write here*]

(b) What further financial resources have become available? From where?

[*Write here*]

11 *Strategies*

Which strategies were chosen to carry out the project and realise the goals? (Several strategies may be specified, guideline examples are mentioned in parentheses.)

( ) (a) Developing/strengthening healthy public policy (e.g. comprehensive non-smoking policy)

[*Write here*]

( ) (b) Developing new laws and regulations (e.g. rules banning smoking in the workplace) by:

[*Write here*]

( ) (c) Reorienting the organisations (e.g. by creating a local public health council) by:

[*Write here*]

( ) (d) Advocating and channelling health interests (e.g. by participating in welfare planning and community development by media advocacy) by:

[*Write here*]

( ) (e) Collaborating and building new alliances (e.g. by bringing together various interested parties by networking) by:

[*Write here*]

( ) (f) Enabling people to change (e.g. by changing the lunch canteen supply, offering exercise during working hours) by:

[*Write here*]

( ) (g) Mobilising/empowering (e.g. by advocating increased direct local influence by groups and people in the area) by:

[*Write here*]

12 Implementation: means and methods

What are the main means used to carry out the project? (Several means may be specified)

( ) Community work
( ) Education/training
( ) Information
( ) Direct lobbying of decision-makers and other key persons
( ) Other (specify)

[*Write here*]

13 Monitoring

What type of continuous monitoring is being done/was done during the project implementation period?

[*Write here*]

14 Evaluation

(a) Completed projects: has the whole project (or parts of it) been evaluated?

( ) Yes   ( ) No

(b) Project in progress: has the whole project (or parts of it) been evaluated?

( ) Yes   ( ) No

(c) Planned projects: Is any evaluation planned?

( ) Yes   ( ) No

(d) If yes, briefly describe how the evaluation has been done/is planned and specify any evaluation documentation

[*Write here*]

15 Impact

(a) What were the short-term results? (for completed projects)

[*Write here*]

(b) What impact has the project had so far? (for projects in progress)

[*Write here*]

16 Outcome

What has been the main long-term outcome?

[*Write here*]

17 Obstacles and solutions

(a) What were the major obstacles/ constraints?

(b) Have they been overcome, and if so, how?

(c) If problems still remain, what are they?

   [*Write here*]

18 Maintenance

What has been done since the project was implemented to ensure that the activities will continue in the future?

[*Write here*]

19 Conclusions for the future

What are the most important conclusions in terms of learning for the future regarding how to renew, reinforce, and/or reorient the activities?

[*Write here*]

20 Documentation

Please list reports, memos, and other documentation of the project/ activities (including media coverage, newspaper articles, videos, etc.)

[*Write here*]

If you have any other comments or information, please write these below:

[*Write here*]

Thanks for Your Contribution!

This questionnaire is to be sent by fax, or E-mail to:
WHO Collaborating Centre on Supportive Environments
Karolinska Institute
Dept of Public Health Sciences
Division of Social Medicine
SE-17176 Stockholm, Sweden
Fax: +46-8-334693

Chapter 6

The development of two instruments to measure the quality of health promotion interventions

Jolanda F.E.M. Keijsers and J.A.M. Saan

INTRODUCTION

More and more attention is being paid to the question: what works in health promotion? Many countries focus on the issue: how to set priorities for health in a more rational way, as budgetary constraints force them to reconsider investment and insurance policies for health. In order to answer that question systematic reviews are conducted. The problem of drawing clear conclusions from publications is in itself difficult, but that is not the focus of this chapter. Published reviews and opinions from articles in journals are not enough to make the conclusions reached productive in practice. What is needed, in addition, is careful translation into guidelines for professionals in the field of health promotion, followed by the development and execution of an implementation strategy.

In this chapter an overview will be given of the health system and policy regarding quality in the Netherlands. Within this context, the Dutch approach is presented, directed on the one hand at reviewing the literature on health promotion effectiveness, and on the other, at translating into guidelines for practitioners. The two key instruments Analys (for analysing the literature) and Preffi (for guiding the professionals) will be discussed and it will be shown that they, in combination, have the potential for continuous and systematic quality improvement in health promotion, including a critical updating of the two instruments themselves.

QUALITY DEVELOPMENT IN THE NETHERLANDS

As in many other countries, the health reform debate has been stimulated by demographic, technological and economic development. Rightly or not, health promotion has been greeted by some as a potential cost-saver, but others have considered it to be another competitor for scarce resources. Criticisms about whether health promotion actually works are often used to undermine the legitimacy of its claims for funding. But questions on effectiveness and efficiency are not only asked of this relative newcomer. As the whole health system starts to copy managerial and administrative methods from the business world, the search is increasing for instruments to guide the process. At the same time, scepticism is increasing regarding the potential of central government to implement relevant policy blue-prints. Quality policy has developed in the context of this leadership crisis.

The concept of quality was introduced to the health system in the 1980s by the medical profession, stimulated by both professional self-criticism and in fear of the American experience of litigation. Focusing on the individual practitioner, training and collaboration were developed. But gradually, taking the example of the quality systems in business, the potential of quality as a core concept in decision-making was recognised.

Quality was seen as a mechanism to keep all parties accountable, to have a rational approach to the development of criteria, to develop feedback mechanisms and to guarantee public access to the data collected. Clarity and comprehensiveness were the values promoted. In the early 1990s several national conferences on health care quality resulted in a three-party agreement between the professions/services, the funds/insurers and the patient organisations. The Ministry of Health acted as a catalyst, not as an active leader. Follow-up was monitored by a national steering committee.

In this committee it became obvious, that, for services like laboratories, ISO systems were very appropriate. However, hospitals adopted an integral approach to quality throughout the whole organisation. General practitioners were developing their identity in competition with hospital based specialists. They took the lead in professional development. They set up a mechanism to establish evidence-based protocols and have linked attendance to post-graduate training, with the renewal of registration. The patient organisations took four years, not only to establish themselves as a platform, but also, to define their role and their own criteria for patient care. The insurance organisations were slowest in adapting quality: they claimed their businesslike nature was guarantee enough and resisted the publication of quality related data, as this would be sensitive information. Their limited involvement is partly due to the variety of insurance organisations: some are general insurance companies with a minor concern for health, others are traditional sick funds, developed from solidarity initiatives.

This 1990 agreement, signed under auspices of the ministry was renewed in 1995. Professional bodies set their own standards and seek to get them adopted/respected by other parties. During 1997 a Society for Quality in Health systems was established, an attempt to harmonise quality systems across organisational boundaries. The Quality Act (Ministry of Health, Welfare and Sport, 1996a) was in operation. This law links developments in health care settings and applies to all of them. The Act requires all organisations to deliver 'responsible care', to have a policy aiming at quality, to have a delineated quality system and to publish an annual report about the quality of care. To enhance the quality of the reports, a national prize has been established.

Responsible care means effective and efficient care at an adequate level which is patient oriented and seeks to meet the real needs of the patient. The law enforces the responsibility of care providers. The Individual Health Care Act applies (Ministry of Health, Welfare and Sport, 1996b) to individual health care professionals.

Health promotion has made major progress through the Public Health Act (Public Health Act, 1990), (which includes health education and health promotion), the realisation of a national network of municipal health services, and the establishment of an infrastructure including the Netherlands Institute for Health Promotion and Disease Prevention (NIGZ). Moreover, a number of specialists are working in the areas of mental health, home care, alcohol and drugs. The Dutch Association for Prevention/Health Education (DAPHE) calculated the number of specialists in 1994 to be 823. Beyond that about 150 specialists work in the ministry and in a number of national organisations and universities.

Initiatives for quality systems are taken mainly by national representative bodies. So most organisations where health promotion specialists work are about to develop or implement quality-systems. In 1992, in keeping with the health system, an Action-program on Quality for Health Promotion was initiated by the NIGZ (Saan, 1993). It sought to make possible the exchange of experience of quality development for health promotion between organisations. Most health organisations were focusing increasingly on the quality of primary processes related to the individual patient. The Action program had three main interdependent areas: professional development, standardisation of work processes and providing an adequate organisational context (see Table 6.1).

Table 6.1 Dutch health promotion quality program

Dutch health promotion quality program Focus	Products
Profession	Charter
	Professional profile
	Ethical code
	Credentialing
	Post-graduate training
	Intervision
Work process	Analys
	Preffi
Organisation	Project management
	Specific criteria built into quality systems

In collaboration with the previously mentioned professional association a charter was developed, i.e. a professional profile with branch-specific sub-profiles (NVPG, 1995). An ethical code is also being discussed. A system of registration, as an entry point to accreditation has been initiated. The quality criteria adopted by the profession have also guided the development of a national training curriculum to be implemented by the Netherlands School of Public Health (Saan, 1996).

The development of the two instruments for health promotion work processes was based on concerns regarding the lack of linkage between research and practice. The research done by universities and other research institutes is not very accessible to practitioners. This is due to the fact that most researchers are interested in models and theories and submit their often technical articles to scientific journals. These journals are not read usually by practitioners, because they do not have the time or skills to do so. A solution could be the wide dissemination of valuable reviews. This can be achieved by standardisation – introducing one standard review method which takes into account all relevant aspects to encourage further quality improvement in health promotion. But even these overviews have their limits. It is better to use standardised reviews to develop guidelines for practitioners, which fit in with the issues and concerns they encounter. Researchers with a focus on design and results, tend to neglect such matters as the political agenda and the limited investment available. Guidelines will enable practitioners to do their work based on the current state of the art in health promotion: 'evidence-based health promotion'. The instruments to enhance the work process will be discussed below.

In the organisational area a standard for project management has been developed. This is implemented initially through a national training program for all specialists working within organisations for the prevention and treatment of alcohol and drugs. Other sections of organisations containing other specialist workers will follow. Most of this work is aimed at fitting relevant health promotion criteria into quality systems as they develop. An example is a standard for the assessment of courses adapted by the home-care organisations.

The Municipal Health Services runs a Quality 2000 program as an external advocacy tool and an internal innovative initiative. Intervision experiments between health educators are part of the process. Home care organisations and alcohol and drug services adapt the ISO approach for their organisations. In mental health prevention, an effort is made to develop national model programmes and have them, after proof of effectiveness, adopted by the regional and local offices.

At present, quality is no longer trendy: case study experiences shared at national conferences show that the long march through the institutions has started. Many health organisations assess quality as perceived and experienced by clients, staff and other stakeholders. They elaborate their models, execute focused projects, and train at least a core group of their personnel. The pioneers have reached the stage of certification, although this is much debated: there is doubt whether it is necessary for all health organisations and who should do it. The prize for the best yearly report slowly gets recognition and helps to stimulate a more serious approach to that tool. In many organisations the Dutch adaptation of the European Quality Award model is being applied, internal auditors are being trained and benchmark reference data becoming available.

If quality policy in the health system is compared to the state of the art within other sectors it is remarkable how quickly this innovation has been adopted and is being implemented. Lessons learned about the technical procedures and problems to be expected during implementation are clearly understood. The rate of adoption is influenced by the context in which this operation takes place. The models for the collection of data are often there, but procedures and information technology are still being tested. Debates about who is responsible and who should pay for this extra system (others, especially government, will debate the 'extra'), and what consequences published data should have, are at an early stage. The role of the Health Inspectorate, who should act on the reports, is being reconsidered accordingly. Another major operation is to reshape the legal position of health professionals and regulate their responsibility; at the same time the legal position of the patient is being reinforced to offer a real power balance; this is also happening in the management of the health organisations.

Few countries take this nationwide approach to quality, linked to the reform of the health system combined with the restructuring of roles of professional and patient. This, in combination with the presence of a recognised body of health promotion specialists, makes the Dutch position better compared to developments in the UK. However, the approach of orchestrating the debate with all actors involved and having government act more as a catalyst is not only limited to the health arena: it is called the Dutch 'polder-model' and is also applied in industry, where employers and unions take co-responsibility for national economic policy.

THE INSTRUMENTS

It is against this context that the development and implementation of the two instruments to standardise work processes will be discussed. They have to be seen as reactions to standardisation. A top-down blue-print approach does not fit with Dutch political and professional culture.

Analys: an instrument for reporting and analysing research

Development

In 1995 the governmental policy paper 'Healthy and Sound' (Ministry of Health, Welfare and Sport, 1995) stated that the estimated potential effectiveness of health promotion as a preventive measure is high. This optimistic judgement was partly based upon the growing number of both national and international review studies. Two problems were encountered when producing two early reviews on effectiveness (Liedekerken *et al.*, 1988; Bosma and

Hosman, 1990). The research design chosen often does not guarantee that clear conclusions can be drawn and the reports often omit data necessary for good comparison with other publications. To enhance the quality of the publications that have to be the building blocks for later reviews, the NIGZ has developed a standard to plan research, to make design decisions and produce useful research reports.

The purpose of a systematic review is to gather and critically appraise all available relevant information related to the effectiveness of a specific intervention. The approach was initially developed to facilitate evidence-based decision-making in clinical medicine (Oxman, 1994). The growing interest in conducting systematic reviews resulted in the foundation of the International Cochrane Collaboration Institute. This worldwide institute comprises thirteen Cochrane centres. The mission of this international network is to prepare, maintain and disseminate systematic reviews of the effects of health care interventions. All relevant data are stored in the Cochrane library. Adapting the Cochrane Collaboration approach to the field of health promotion leads to a number of problems. One of them is the fact that within health promotion the variety of intervention processes is large, so it is very important to gather detailed information about the nature of the intervention and use that information to interpret the results found. Already several countries have begun attempts to compile evidence of effectiveness for health promotion interventions. However, different review methods are used and only now databases are being developed in which all the information is stored in an accessible way, for example, the EPI-centre London UK (Peersman *et al.*, 1996).

Based on experiences of an early effort to establish such a database in 1986, the Netherlands Institute for Health Promotion and Disease Prevention developed a checklist on the basis of which intervention studies in health promotion can be analysed (Driel and Keijsers, 1997). There were two reasons for developing it. First, there was no standard and nationally agreed checklist available for analysing the literature on effectiveness studies in health promotion. Second, to increase the knowledge of what is effective in health promotion, a clearer and more detailed way of reporting evaluated health promotion interventions was needed.

Research in the area of health promotion shows that a carefully planned intervention is more likely to be effective. This is highlighted by the model which strongly emphasises the systematical implementation and monitoring of the planning and evaluation process (Kok, 1992). During the planning process five questions need to be answered: (1) how serious is the problem?; (2) what behaviour and whose behaviour is involved?; (3) what are the determinants of the behaviour?; (4) which intervention can change the behaviour and its determinants?; and (5) how can the developed intervention be implemented? The evaluation process in the model implies the assessment of the success of the intervention changing behaviour and its behavioural determinants. The model is presented in Figure 6.1.

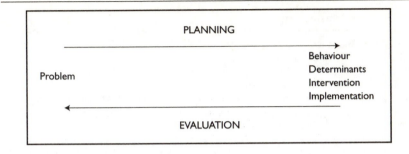

Figure 6.1 The planning and evaluation process of health promotion

The central items of the review instrument (Analys) were based on this model. At the same time effectiveness criteria from other sources were borrowed. An example of a so-called effect condition is 'feedback'. From the work of Mullen *et al.* (1985), it can be concluded that the provision of information to the learner and learning about his/her accomplishments is an important condition for an intervention being effective.

Description of the instrument

The review instrument (Analys) distinguishes eight themes, which are sub-divided into 39 criteria in total, phrased as multiple choice questions. Answering these questions yields insight into: (1) the methodological quality of a study; (2) the effects of an intervention; and (3) the process by which this effect was achieved. The latter is important because it provides information that could explain the effects found. The instrument also contains a glossary and an instruction. In Table 6.2 the outline of Analys is given.

Applying Analys in the above described way will lead to clear and systematic reviews. This implies that, compared to the traditional review, the reader gains a better understanding of how the information was gathered and analysed so that the interpretations and conclusions can be checked. Furthermore, by applying Analys, detailed information on the nature of the intervention will be gathered. This is important for further insight into what makes health promotion work.

Implementation and use

Analys was pretested in several settings, revised and then accepted in a national consensus meeting. The International Union for Health Promotion and Health Education (IUHPE) then used Analys to review international literature concerning the effectiveness of health promotion interventions (IUHPE/Euro, 1995). The feedback, provided by colleagues from very different backgrounds and its application in a number of topics, was very helpful.

Table 6.2 Global format Analys

Global format Analys Themes	Questions related to
Problem	Size and severity
Target group	Mean age, number of men/women, level of education, income
Behaviour	Causal relations, determinants of the behaviour, type of behaviour
Target	Targets of the intervention
Intervention	Development and execution of the intervention, use of theories, type of intervention, specific content of the intervention, phase of the intervention, place of execution of the intervention, previous experience with the execution of the intervention, duration of the intervention, participation to the intervention
Implementation	Anticipation to broader use of the intervention
Process evaluation	Type of research methods, type of data, satisfaction with the intervention, type of recommendations based on the process evaluation
Effect evaluation	Size of the research population, selection of the research population, comparability of research groups, method of effect evaluation, measurements, percentage dropouts, reach of the intervention, effect parameters, fit between effects found and targets stated

Analys is not only useful for stimulating clear review reports and retrospectively analysing the literature. It can be a check on detailed processes and comprehensiveness for others to judge research proposals and articles. We encountered a readiness to adopt the idea, but a resistance to use it systematically in its present format when interviewing editors of professional journals. Editorial work is often a voluntary job and using Analys would perhaps make the life of writers and editors more effective, but not easier. National funding organisations understood the benefit of judging proposals more systematically and even considered requiring systematic applications, using the proposed format. The National Research and Development Council for Health is using Analys as an integral part of their own criteria to describe, assess and report.

Preffi: an instrument for guiding practitioners

Development

It has already been noted that even the most clearly analysed articles might not reach the practitioner. A system of transfer and linkage is required. Integrative guidelines for practitioners had to be developed based upon the results of systematic reviews. Although evidence from research is an essential input for practice guidelines, it is not sufficient. The guidelines should be interpreted in the light of users' preferences and the (health care) setting in which the recommendations are implemented (Cook *et al.*, 1997). This implies that issues like feasibility and finance are also of importance.

Preffi is the abbreviation of health PRomotion EFfectiveness Fostering Instrument. The Preffi was developed in close consultation with researchers and practitioners. It was introduced at a national conference and is available as a place-mat (a double-sided, plastic coated A4 leaflet) to stress its ready-to-use features. Nowadays it could be a mouse-mat. (An English version is available.)

Description of the instrument

Preffi is also based on the model of planning and evaluating health education indicated in Figure 6.1. Consequently, Analys and Preffi have comparable formats, which in turn fit with the established academic training that many specialists receive now.

As well as the necessity of working on the basis of the above mentioned model, special attention is paid within Preffi to its organisational and managerial opportunities in practice. Issues in this respect include conditions, project management and implementation requirements. The global format of Preffi is presented in Table 6.3.

Table 6.3 Global format Preffi

Global format Preffi Themes	Three central questions
Context/conditions	1 How much attention is paid to these topics?
Nature and scope of problem	
(Behavioural) determinants	2 How in future can this be improved?
Target group	
Target	3 What are the priorities for improvement?
Intervention	
Effective elements build into the intervention	
Project management	
Pretest	
Execution/implementation	
Process and effect evaluation	

Several aspects are included under every theme. Under the theme 'target group', for instance, the following features are mentioned: general characteristics of target group, specific characteristics of segments of target groups and inventories of their needs, wishes and choices.

In order to improve the quality of health promotion in practice, practitioners need to point out how much attention is paid to each of these aspects and how in future this can be improved. Furthermore, priorities should be set, for everything can not be done simultaneously. All these monitoring activities should finally result in a plan directed at quality improvement.

Implementation and use

All items are explained in the guidelines to the instrument. Suggestions for its use are given, based on pretests. At present the degree of spontaneous uptake is being assessed as part of a three year implementation strategy, supported by monitoring research. Conditions for further implementation are being discussed. The strategy includes training of specialists, exchanging case studies, and a Preffi Prize which is given to exceptional examples of its use. A revised version will emanate from these experiences.

The instruments in combination

Analys and Preffi should not be considered in isolation. Their use in combination, as illustrated in Figure 6.2, provides a systematic, coherent development directed to evidence-based health promotion (Keijsers *et al.*, 1996). Figure 6.2 shows that the system is bridging the gap between research and practice by summarising and incorporating the results of research into guidelines and assisting practitioners in their work in everyday practice. The higher the quality of the research done, the more effectively the results are clearly interpreted and translated into conclusions and the more evidence-based the guidelines will be. On the other hand, practitioners are requested to make monitoring and research a common element in their work. Their experiences may help to suggest new hypotheses to be tested and will challenge the old criteria used so far. Additional evidence will be utilised and adapted to produce new guidelines for practice.

Another issue illustrated in Figure 6.2 is that implementation is a separate and thus explicit phase in the whole process. Both instruments should be implemented based on a careful examination of the several stages a person goes through before he or she is working with the instrument as a routine activity (Rogers, 1995).

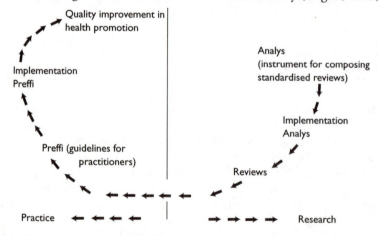

Figure 6.2 Quality improvement in health promotion

Finally, it should be noted, that this is an iterative process with two spin-offs. Like most quality processes it is aiming at two improvements: not only of the research and practice, but also of the instruments themselves.

Changing practice

Some research is published on how guidelines can be disseminated and implemented in such a way that practitioners are really acting upon them and thus changing their behaviour. A lot of the research originates from medical practice (e.g. Grimshaw and Russel, 1993). Within the Cochrane network a special review group aims to help bridge the gap between evidence of the effects of health care and the delivery of effective and efficient care by preparing and maintaining systematic reviews of the effects and costs of interventions that influence professional practice. This group is called the Cochrane Collaboration of Effective Professional Practice (CCEPP). The reviews prepared by this group are very useful for health promotion since they will provide information on what works in changing practitioners' behaviour. Currently, a review is being prepared on how health professionals could be kept up to date with evidence derived from sound research. With that perspective the effectiveness of educational meetings or workshops and the effectiveness of audit and feedback in improving practice are studied (Thomson, 1997).

Changing research

Currently Preffi is being implemented on a large scale. Experiences with it will not only help to improve the criteria for practice, but suggest other criteria to enhance the relevance of research. Alongside 'evidence-based health promotion practice' 'practice based research' will develop. Experience is being acquired, both with systematic proposal assessment and with dissemination of research/results by the National Research and Development Council on Health. The investment in research is also being judged by the opportunities of guaranteeing implementability on a larger scale at a later stage. Rational programming of research and its use is gaining ground.

DUTCH QUALITY DEVELOPMENT IN PERSPECTIVE

A well-known law in health promotion states: health knowledge does not lead to behaviour change. Now we have to face, that professional knowledge alone does not lead to improved quality without targeted, systematic action. All these efforts make one conclusion obvious: professionals, both researchers and practitioners, behave like normal people.

The use of both instruments requires implementation effort. Therefore the link with two areas in quality policy, professional development and organisational context (including project management as standard for organisational processes) is crucial. Not only should these instruments be taught at all universities that prepare health promotion specialists. It is important to stimulate practice to adopt these models for case/analysis. On the other hand, integration in organisation-wide quality systems is necessary. Many services are updating their management information using information technology. It can be crucial at that stage to make sure that the units selected to make health promotion account for its actions, fit with the principles and processes covered by these instruments.

A challenge will be to balance between the simple type of checklists and the variety of criteria generated by increasing knowledge. It is tempting to overestimate the readiness to change within the profession. So the linkage between these instruments, the professionalism of the users and the organisational context has to be ensured. Quality talk may be misused to add another layer of professional jargon, that is part of the fence any professional group tends to erect around its domain (Saan, 1997). In keeping with the health promotion principle of equitable public access to policy and strategy for health, instruments like these should aim at making the professional's work clear and accessible. Accountability and responsibility foster public dialogue, if a professional group seeks to answer to all stakeholders involved. Quality is a shared form of self-criticism, based upon the starting point that only the dissatisfied are ready for change.

The Netherlands has three major assets to facilitate the use of these quality instruments. The political and organisational context is positive. 'Quality' and 'evidence' are considered key phrases in health systems reform. The search is on for ways and means that involve all parties in steering the health system, as the political power to intervene in the rising costs have failed so far: politicians don't like to cut health spending: it may cost votes.

The second advantage is the relatively small scale of the country and the intensity with which sharing of learning about quality takes place. The emerging quality specialists are a thriving force in this development. In hospitals quality is also a tool in the battle between management and medical specialists about who controls what. Both try to apply the quality debate for that purpose. In pharmacies, an innovative project on quality started and experiences from other settings were transferred to create the contours of that quality program: sharing experiences strengthens implementation.

Finally, focusing on health promotion, the availability of a nationwide network of specialists and organisations leading in health promotion programs make the Dutch situation comparable to the setting in the UK. An intensive sharing of strategic approaches and experiences with this country is being sought. The very existence of the NIGZ as an institute whose core business, next to health oriented interventions is the linkage between policy, research and practice, is a critical context to guarantee long-term investment in development and use of these types of instruments. National institutes in other countries are a natural colleague and partner. The IUHPE project offered an opportunity to extend the exchange across Europe and confirmed the impression that the number of fortunate conditions specified here contribute to the impact quality policy will have on health promotion, not only in the Netherlands. We expect those conditions to assist in further elaboration and improvement of the instruments discussed. This book is part of the bridge we want to build.

References

Bosma, M. and C. Hosman (1990), *Preventie op waarde geschat* (Mental Health Promotion Effectiveness; in Dutch) Nijmegen: Beta Boeken.

Cook, D.J., Greengold, N.L., Ellrodt, A.G. and Weingarten, S.R. (1997). The relation between systematic reviews and practical guidelines. *Annals of Internal Medicine* 3: 210–216.

Driel, W.G. van and Keijsers, J.F.E.M. (1997). An instrument for reviewing the effectiveness of health education and health promotion. *Patient Education and Counseling*, 30: 7–17.

Grimshaw, J.M. and Russell, I.T. (1993). Effect of clinical guidelines on medical practice: a systematic review of rigorous evaluations. *Lancet* 342: 1,317–1,322.

IUHPE/Euro (1995). *An Instrument for Analyzing Effectiveness Studies on Health Promotion and Health Education* (including 16 publications on topics). Woerden: International Union for Health Promotion and Health Education,

Keijsers, J.F.E.M., Molleman, G.M.R. and van Driel, W.G. (1996). *Reviewing and Guiding the Effectiveness of Behavioral Health Promotion*. Third European Conference on Quality Assessment, Torino.

Kok, G.J. (1992). Quality of planning as a decisive determinant of health education effectiveness. *Hygie* 11: 5–8.

Liedekerken, P., Jonkers, R. *et al.* (1988). *The Effectiveness of Health Education*, Rijswijk: Uitgeverij voor Gezondheidsbevordering.

Ministry of Health, Welfare and Sport (1995). *Healthy and Sound*. Rijswijk.

Ministry of Health, Welfare, and Sport (1996a). De Kwaliteitswet en de Wet BIG (The Quality Act and the Individual Health Care Professions Act), *Nieuwsbrief De Wet BIG* 5: 6–7.

Ministry of Health, Welfare, and Sport (1996b). *Factsheet Quality Act in Care-organizations*. Rijswijk (English version).

Mullen, P.D., Green, L.W. and Persinger, G.S. (1985). Clinical trials of patient education for chronic conditions: a comparative meta-analysis of intervention types. *Preventive Medicine* 14: 753–781.

NVPG (1995) *Beroepsprofiel 1995–1997* (Professional Charter and Profile; in Dutch), NVPG/LCG.

Oxman, A.D. (ed.) (1994). *The Cochrane Collaboration Handbook*. Oxford: Cochrane Collaboration.

Peersman, G., Oliver, S. *et al.* (1996) *Establishing an Information, Resource and Training Centre on Evidence Based Health Promotion*. Third European Conference on Quality Assessment, Torino.

Rogers, E.M. (1995). *Diffusion of Innovations*. Fourth revised edition. New York: The Free Press.

Saan, J.A.M. (1993) *Actieprogramman Kwaliteit* (Actionprogram Quality). LCG.

Saan, J.A.M. (1996) *Postdoctoraal Onderwijs Gezondheid en gedrag* (Dutch text of a national postgraduate curriculum). Woerden: NIGZ

Saan, J.A.M. (1997) Quality revisited. *Promotion & Education*, 4, 2: 34–35.

Thomson, M.A. (1997). *Decisions and reviews about continuing education and quality assurance*. Abstract Book, Second International Conference on the Scientific Basis of Health Services. Amsterdam, 5–8 October.

Chapter 7

Quality assessment in health promotion settings

Viv Speller, Liz Rogers and Annette Rushmere

In the 1990s health promotion practice has had to respond rapidly to policy initiatives and changes in health care organisation and funding. The impact on practitioners of health promotion has been substantial both in changing ways of working and thinking about their roles and the impact they have on health. Whilst this had led to some demonstrable and arguably positive changes in practice, it has not been without threat and uncertainty. In the UK these influences have been particularly evident as the health care system within which many health promoters work changed fundamentally in the wake of the health care reforms. These changes were characterised most sharply by the organisational separation of purchasers and providers of health care (DOH, 1989), a division which has not led to any consistent pattern of organisational arrangements for health promotion services in the UK; and subsequently by the emphasis placed on researching the evidence base of health care through the establishment of wide-ranging mechanisms for influencing the direction and financing of health services research (DOH, 1991). These twin drivers have affected the development of quality assessment in health promotion in different ways. This chapter will seek to explore the influence of these policy drivers on quality assessment in health promotion in the UK, and to draw lessons for the wider practice of health promotion from reflections on the experience of health promoters and changes in their practice over recent years. It will do so by examining five quality assessment schemes developed by the Wessex Institute for Health Research and Development in the south of England in the 1990s. Each of these schemes was developed for a different health promotion setting or group of practitioners, has been implemented widely and is still in use.

Reflection on the development of quality assurance in health care and health promotion suggests that there are five key elements that may be important in describing approaches to quality. There are two main styles of quality assurance: the approach closer to that used in industry, External Standards Inspection (ESI) where standards are set, applied to a work process, monitored and action taken if standards are not met; and Total Quality Management (TQM) or the similar process of Continuous Quality Improvement (CQI). Examples of ESI in health care would include performance standards for waiting times in clinics or maximum ambulance arrival times. There have been many descriptions of TQM/CQI approaches which are characterised by a change in management culture, training in quality issues and internal derivation of quality processes and standards (Joss and Kogan, 1995). The key distinctions between the styles are: internal versus external standards setting; and a sense of quality assurance as continuous growth rather than maintaining a static service meeting minimum performance levels.

Quality can also be considered from different perspectives with sometimes conflicting requirements and expectations. Thus Ovretveit (1992) suggests three dimensions of client, professional and management quality, which need to be integrated in order to specify the quality of a particular service. For health promotion the dimension of client may be harder to assess as this might include the wider community as well as a service user, the term 'consumer' is used to include both direct recipients of service and the wider community (Ovretveit, 1996). Thus the five key elements appear to concern the balance between internal and external standards of quality in health promotion and how to assess them; and who defines those standards, be they professional health promoters or other stakeholders, management, i.e. purchasers or funding bodies, and consumers who use or are influenced by the health promotion activity. These five elements will be applied as a yardstick to the following projects to see how far they match up and to identify any shortcomings.

A further typology of quality assurance will also be applied. We have found it helpful to consider approaches in terms of whether they are a 'quality assurance programme', that is an attempt to apply quality assurance principles to all aspects of a department or service's activities; or a 'quality initiative', a scheme or settings-based programme that is in some way quality assured. Whilst the distinction is not always absolute, for example a quality initiative may be a step on the way to developing a service-wide approach, it does help to distinguish those approaches which attempt to provide an overall framework and culture for quality assurance. Finally we will consider whether any of the schemes have been evaluated and what impact they appear to have had. The five schemes are: a project to develop quality assurance for the generic practice of health promotion specialists; a tool for planning, evaluating and developing healthy alliances; a Healthy School Award; an organisational approach to developing Health Promoting Hospitals, and a Healthy Leisure Award.

QUALITY ASSURANCE FOR HEALTH PROMOTION SPECIALISTS IN THE NHS

The Health Education Authority for England commissioned the Wessex Institute to develop 'relevant and accessible' quality assurance methods for health promotion specialists in 1993. The project took twelve months and aimed to provide practitioners with a theoretical and operational framework as well as model standards and criteria for adaptation to local need. A manual providing guidance on quality assurance concepts and methods, characteristics of good practice in health promotion, model standards and criteria and practical assistance with starting a quality assurance programme was produced (Evans *et al.*, 1994; Speller *et al.*, 1997). The project was initially proposed by an advisory team of purchasers and providers of health promotion, in order to provide means by which purchasers could contract for specified programmes of activity and monitor progress against agreed objectives. Around this time there were early examples of competitive tendering for the provision of health promotion services. Some practitioners felt it was necessary to have a more explicit and objective way of demonstrating their abilities to deliver high quality health promotion in the face of competition from other providers. Thus the context in which this project was undertaken was one of 'tooling up' health promotion to fit in the new climate of the contract culture and it was therefore firmly rooted in the NHS arena and focused solely on the roles of health promotion specialists employed by the NHS, although many aspects of their work were conducted in other settings.

Consultation took place throughout the life of the project, and draft materials were widely circulated at each stage of development. The project was advertised nationally to seek examples of good practice in quality assurance or audit from health promotion departments. Individuals identified by this process gave advice and case studies were included in the final document. Structured discussions were held with managers and staff of health promotion services in five health service regions in England and Wales, and piloting of draft standards was supported by teams in the local area. These discussions centred around consideration of definitions of quality assurance and descriptions of processes as derived from the literature and other professional practice, and the characteristics of good practice as perceived by the profession. This consensus approach ensured that the definitions, standards and methods conformed to current health promotion practice, rather than to theoretical ideals. Thus in terms of the three dimensions of quality described above, this approach took account of management and professional definitions of quality. Although aspects of the measures described referred to processes for assessing consumer satisfaction with services, the perspective of the wider community dimension was lacking in development.

The manual outlined six key functions of health promotion: strategic planning; programme management; monitoring and evaluation; education and training; resources and information and advice and consultancy. Twenty-five model standards and 106 measurable criteria were proposed, with guidelines for assessment. Importantly although these standards were presented as core measures of quality, it was recognised that a generic framework such as this could not encompass the detail of specific types of programmes relating to settings and topics in different contexts. Thus additional guidance was given on processes for teamwork, both to introduce quality assurance concepts to the department and to derive locally adapted standards. This was therefore a framework for department-wide quality assurance programmes, that was developed internally by the profession. It did however also provide some milestones that could be considered as minimum professional standards that could then be applied externally whilst leaving room for further tailoring at the level of local teams.

Following publication the manual was given a high profile through a national launch and distribution to all NHS health promotion services in England. However, further dissemination was *ad hoc*, there were presentations at various conferences and training events, and some use of clinical audit funds to encourage its application. In June 1996 a national postal survey of the development of quality assurance in specialist health promotion services in England was carried out (Royle and Speller, 1996). The survey aimed to: assess the current state of practice in quality assurance in health promotion in England; the impact that the manual had had on practice; what processes or methods practitioners were using; and what further support they required. The response rate was 70 per cent, and nearly all the respondents (92 per cent) had seen a copy of the manual and most had used it in some way to shape their quality assurance programmes, over half of the respondents had quality assurance programmes running in their departments. Most respondents felt that internal peer review was the best way to monitor standards, with correspondingly few supporting external audit. However, views were equally split on whether or not there should be a common set of national standards and criteria for assuring quality in health promotion, with about a third agreeing, disagreeing and undecided respectively. Practitioners indicated that they would welcome further training on quality assurance, and that time and resources would facilitate implementation of quality assurance programmes. It thus appears that this project effectively engaged health promotion practitioners in quality assurance and had an impact on the way they work. This was influenced by the wide availability of the materials nationally, and by the accessibility and relevance of the methods and standards proposed.

EVALUATING HEALTHY ALLIANCES

The concept of intersectoral working was given new impetus in England by the health strategy, the Health of the Nation (DOH, 1992), which stressed the importance of bringing together different sectors in the pursuit of targets for improved public health. In the context of a performance managed health service, alliances needed to be accountable and to assess the effectiveness of investments in services or particular interventions. A project was funded between 1993 and 1995 by the HEA to develop a framework for agreeing indicators of success of health alliance work that could be adapted to local needs and objectives. This resulted in the publication of a manual for alliance workers to use in assessing both the processes and outputs of their activities in a practical manner (Funnell *et al.*, 1995). The first year of the project was spent developing an initial set of measures to evaluate the effectiveness of healthy alliances. Participation from alliance practitioners from all sectors was considered essential, both to learn from their wealth of experience and to shape a product that would meet users' needs. This involved over 200 people in three stages: a telephone survey to identify examples of good practice in alliance evaluation; second, workshops with respondents selected on the basis of evaluation experience debated what were considered to be characteristics of successful alliances and what measures they used. These discussions were analysed qualitatively using the words and concepts illustrated in the discussions to form two sets of indicators of processes and outputs of alliance work. Third, a consensus forum was held with a wider group of participants and stakeholders in healthy alliances for critical examination of the indicators. It was notable that the terminology used in the draft at this stage was that of quality assurance, indicators being presented as standards and criteria, but this was not felt to be helpful by participants and was dropped in the final version. A consensus was reached about the content and shape of the final draft pack which was then tested in five case studies of alliances for a further year.

The field testing aimed to assess the acceptability and generalisability of the indicators across both alliances and different types of projects. Support was provided to alliance teams to familiarise them with the pack and to implement an evaluation. At the end of the testing period focus groups and a questionnaire were used to collect feedback from participants, and all those who had requested the draft materials during the year were also surveyed. A consultation workshop was also held for health service purchasers. The pack was rewritten in the light of all comments received providing an evaluation framework of eleven categories of process and output indicators (see Table 7.1). The process indicators are: commitment; community participation; communication; joint working and accountability. Each is presented in a checklist format of detailed indicators for each category. The output indicators covered six categories of types of output of alliance work: policy change; service and environment change; skills development; publicity; contact and change in knowledge, attitude or behaviour. As the objectives and content of projects will vary tremendously between and within alliances, a checklist of questions to consider was given to enable groups to define specific indicators in the category that are applicable to their particular situation.

This process combined both management and professional views of quality, and was internally derived with a very strong emphasis on user involvement and ownership of the final format. Once again the dimension of consumer involvement was less clear. The consultation included representatives from non-statutory sectors and in some of the test sites the evaluation was undertaken by project groups including community members. These examples illuminated problems with the language and perspective of the draft materials which were

Table 7.1 Process and output indicator statements from 'Towards Healthier Alliances'

Process Indicators	Statement
Commitment	The partners are committed to the goals of the alliance, holding a shared vision of what the group can contribute and gain as a whole and as individuals. They are open and honest in this respect. The appropriate people are involved in the alliance and the participants have the necessary skills and experience. Other necessary resources are identified and each partner contributes what they can to these.
Community Involvement	The alliance involves the community in all its activities, including agenda-setting, planning, decision-making and operational activities. There is community representation within the membership with the necessary training and skills. The representatives feel that they have an equal stake in the alliance. The community has a voice that is listened to and respected.
Communication	The alliance has effective two-way communication between the participants and between them and partner organisations. It encourages 'networking' at all levels. This is underpinned by simplicity, honesty and openness. The alliance ensures that the public has access to information about the alliance and its activity. It has a strategy to accept and respond to information or requests for information from the wider community, and has given attention to its public and corporate image.
Joint working	The alliance partners work together as a team to produce joint strategies and action plans and seek opportunities to develop new areas of work together. Joint work implies ownership and appropriate input from each partner.
Accountability	Alliance members are fully accountable and can provide justification for their actions to each other, to parent organisations and to the wider community. Each member takes responsibility for this. Evaluation is built into alliance work and the results are used constructively.

Output Indicators	Statement
Policy change	The alliance aims to establish new policies or change existing ones which promote, protect or maintain health. It has clear aims for the level of change to be achieved within appropriate timescales. The quality of the policies has been considered. Policies are monitored to ensure that any changes meet their criteria and have been put into practice. The alliance observes any resulting effect on the target group, and looks for unintended results. Future objectives are set in the light of the successes and problems encountered.
Service and environment change	The alliance aims to help establish environmental, organisational, service or structural changes which may affect the target group. It has clear aims and has set appropriate timescales for achieving these. The alliance monitors the results and observes any effects on the target group. Successes and problems are considered and any unanticipated results observed. New objectives are set in the light of these.

Table 7.1 continued

Output Indicators	Statement
Skills development	The alliance provides or arranges the provision of training and skills development for the target group and for partner organisations of the alliance which is monitored to ensure that attendance is appropriate and reasons for non-attendance explored. The effects of the training are observed and needs are continually assessed.
Publicity	The alliance actively makes use of opportunities to give public information or publicity about alliance activities. Coverage through these efforts and unplanned coverage is assessed to monitor how much publicity it has achieved and the quality. Opportunities to respond to it are taken. The alliance ensures that the coverage reaches the intended audience whenever possible and reviews this accordingly.
Contact	The alliance maximises direct contact between the target group and alliance activities. There are clear aims and objectives, and targets are set within appropriate timescales. The alliance monitors contact and the results of the activity are observed, including unanticipated effects. Successes and problems are considered and new objectives set in the light of these where necessary.
Knowledge, attitude and behaviour change	The alliance aims to affect the target group's knowledge, attitudes and behaviour. It has considered ways of determining measures of these before activity begins and has set clear objectives for change. The alliance observes any changes, making use of indicators where possible. The extent of detail will depend on resources and support available.

amended in the final version, highlighting the importance of including the consumer dimension in agreeing measures of quality. The approach taken in this project rested firmly within the TQM or CQI model. The guidance was predicated on the twin assumptions that good quality of management of the alliance processes will yield more effective outputs; and that alliances are at very different stages of development and will learn and grow from evaluating themselves. Much of the emphasis in the presentation was to provide assistance with methods of reflection on work practice and its assessment, through exercises and step by step guidance. The framework enables an alliance to develop a quality assurance programme for its work, although it recognised that this may need to be introduced in stages.

Subsequently 'Towards Healthier Alliances' has been widely used by alliances in the UK and the WHO Healthy Cities Project, and provided the evaluation criteria to judge the English 'Health Alliance Award Scheme' which was run annually by the Department of Health to encourage alliance working in the key areas covered by the Health of the Nation. It was also used by the Health Education Board for Scotland and ASH Scotland to evaluate and provide guidance for smoking cessation alliances in Scotland, and was found to be a robust and useful framework (Duffy, 1997).

AN AUDIT AND ACCREDITATION TOOL FOR HEALTH PROMOTING HOSPITALS

The Health Promoting Hospital (HPH) initiative with its emphasis on health gain through health promotion provides a vehicle for secondary care providers to contribute to the Health of the Nation targets. Guidance on developing Health Promoting Hospitals was sent out widely to the NHS by the NHS Executive (DOH, 1994). In the south and west of England this was presented to representatives from hospitals and health promotion services at a conference in Salisbury in December 1994. When asked what support participants would require in implementing the initiative they strongly urged that a more systematic approach should be taken to develop standards for health promoting hospitals to move beyond the rhetoric to achievable and measurable changes in hospital services. A management group of purchasers and providers was established to develop a practical tool that would assist the development of HPH. The group decided to develop an audit tool based on a self-assessment audit framework for purchasers that had been locally developed. This document consisted of key areas each with detailed criteria, and organisations were encouraged to make comments and reference key documents required for evidence of meeting the criteria. A total organisational approach was taken for the HPH audit tool including review of existing quality initiatives and other current NHS initiatives that impacted on the health care of patients, the health of staff and the internal and external environment of the hospital. Links with primary care, social services and other agencies were also included along with other community links with local alliances, schools and industry. The final audit tool consists of six key areas that relate to aspects of the organisation's functions with associated measurable criteria (Rushmere, 1997). These are: management issues; customer care; healthy workplaces; hotel services and environmental issues; community and health alliances; clinical audit and effectiveness. The key statements relating to each of these are presented in Table 7.2. These six elements include all the current quality initiatives required of hospitals in the NHS in England, incorporating them in a single framework and ensuring that the health promoting elements of each are emphasised.

This audit tool and accreditation process was developed by hospital managers and staff in collaboration with purchasers. It is thus clearly identifiable as an internally derived tool incorporating the perspectives of managers and professionals. Again, whilst elements encompassed by the tool include areas where customer satisfaction measures are paramount, its development process did not include the participation of service users. Whilst its objectives are to assess performance across each of the six areas noting strengths and areas for improvement, the standards are explicit and the process of audit includes external assessment by peers. It therefore combines elements of the TQM and ESI approaches to quality assurance. It is an example of a settings-based, rather than generic, quality assurance programme providing an organisational

Table 7.2 Key areas and statements from the Health Promoting Hospitals audit and accreditation tool

Key area	Statement
Management issues	Central to the success of this project is a strategic approach which involves the staff, patients, visitors and the community. The project should demonstrate a long-term vision of healthcare that recognises the shift of focus from treating illness and disease to maintaining good health and promoting health and well-being.
Customer care	In this section the customer is defined as the patient and the carer. Organisations should be able to demonstrate that they have user involvement in the planning and implementation of services. Systems should reflect the view that users have comprehensive information about services. Organisations should be able to demonstrate that they have a commitment to the communication of information to patients and carers to support shared decision-making and awareness of their own care. Organisations should also be committed to equal opportunities and ethnic minority issues relating to patients and carers using their services.
Healthy workplaces	This section is related to staff and the workplace. Organisations should be able to demonstrate that they have a commitment and an ongoing plan to support and promote health in the workplace. Organisations should also be committed to promoting equal opportunities for present and future employees. It is in the interest of an organisation as well as in the interest of its employees to utilise the skills of the total workforce.
Hotel services and environmental issues	Organisations should be able to demonstrate a strategic approach towards the implementation of national guidelines for nutrition and British and European standards for hotel and environmental services. They should be able to demonstrate a commitment to improving the organisation's environment for its customers and staff both internally and externally and in developing 'green' policies.
Community and health alliances	Organisations should be able to demonstrate a strategic approach to community involvement and alliance partnerships that moves beyond the seeking of community views to active involvement by the community with the hospital. Clarity about what is intended in the form of clear objectives should be supported by specific measures of how progress will be achieved. In addition organisations should be able to share the vision to inform longer-term relationships.
Clinical audit and effectiveness	Decisions made by hospitals should be informed by a wide variety of research and intelligence from clinical audit that embraces health needs and clinical effectiveness. Health improvement through effective targeting of clinical interventions and health promotion activities which reflect HON priorities are essential. This requires a better understanding about relationships between treatment and outcomes. Local action should be informed by use of knowledge generated from a wide variety of sources, including research and development and a range of other national initiatives.

umbrella for the assessment and development of quality initiatives in different areas of hospital service.

The tool was evaluated to ascertain impressions of the process and the impacts it had on organisations through interviews conducted with board level hospital managers, by a researcher who had not been involved in the development process. Providers noted benefits of the scheme such as: 'the audit process triggers and accelerates change'; 'It has embedded health promotion into the culture of organisations' and 'It raised awareness of health promotion and helped to change attitudes'. Purchasers noted that the tool: 'provides a framework for discussion and gives a focus for negotiating Health of the Nation'; 'provides a detailed picture of qualitative activity within a Trust, particularly an Acute trust' and 'action plans could be translated into contracts and monitored year on year'. The peer review process, whereby purchasers, managers and non-executive directors from one Trust paid review visits to another as part of the accreditation process, was particularly welcomed and served to exchange good practice between organisations to improve quality. The tool is being used in health authorities in the South and West region, and resulting action plans for trusts have been incorporated into their service contracts to ensure continuity and monitoring of progress.

THE WESSEX HEALTHY SCHOOLS AWARD

The Wessex Healthy Schools Award was developed in 1992 by an alliance of health professionals, education advisers and pilot schools in four counties in the south of England (Rogers *et al.*, 1993). It is a systematic approach to school based health promotion, offering schools an opportunity to develop a focus and a framework for cross-curricular planning and delivery of health education. Seventeen schools, including both primary and secondary schools (age 5–18 years) took part in the development process, devising appropriate statements of success and methods of implementation. In addition local health promotion departments and education authority inspectors and advisers were closely involved.

The scheme encompasses change in three broad areas: school curriculum content; school culture and environment; and interaction between the school and the home and wider community. It enables schools to build on existing work towards becoming a health-promoting school, identifies areas where progress could be made and sets targets for improvement which are monitored two to three terms later to validate achievement of the award. The scheme was developed by the regional health authority as part of a national 'Look After Your Heart' programme alongside other heart disease prevention initiatives in workplaces and community settings. It was felt to be an attractive way of committing schools to a comprehensive programme of health promotion that extended beyond the curriculum. At the time the financing and management arrangements for schools were changing giving individual schools more responsibility for marketing themselves and managing their own budgets. The emphasis on an award, a recognised level of achievement of standards approved by the Education Authority, was therefore seen as a means of gaining recognition for the school's work in this regard, and presenting a caring image to prospective parents. The links with school inspection were enhanced by the validation visits which were conducted by an 'Ofsted' inspector (Office for Standards in Education) with expertise in personal, social and health education. The value placed on the Healthy Schools Award by schools is demonstrated by the way in which they frequently use evidence collected for the achievement of the award in their regular full Ofsted inspections. Given the contract culture in the NHS, the award also allowed purchasers to contract for joint funded work with education authorities of a specified volume (target numbers of schools engaged) to a predetermined standard (achievement of the award).

The award identifies nine key statements of standards that are expected of a health-promoting school covering: national curriculum; wider community; smoke-free environment; nutrition; physical activity; responsibility for health; staff health; environment and equal opportunities (Table 7.3). Schools receive a booklet describing these and a development planner to help them plan their approach. An initial visit by an education authority adviser, or NHS health promotion specialist, helps the school identify the two areas they will concentrate on for validation and assesses a baseline position. During the course of the year the local health promotion specialists provide training and individual support to schools to help them achieve the changes, and a resource pack provides suggestions on types of activities in each area. An Ofsted inspector validates the school at the end of the year by assessing the progress made. Generally, education authorities and health authorities jointly organise award ceremonies where the participating schools in their area receive their award from the chief executives of the authorities, and celebrate their achievement through displays of their work, usually involving children as well as staff and supporters. In 1997 there were approximately 300 schools participating in the award scheme, many of them being revalidated for a second and third year.

This scheme was one of the first to be developed in this style in the UK. We were interested to examine the extent to which the approach had been adopted elsewhere, and what form any other schemes took. We conducted a survey of all health promotion units in the UK in 1996; 66 per cent responded (Rogers *et al.*, 1998). Of these half (51 per cent) were involved with a similar joint health and education scheme and a fifth (21 per cent) were planning one. Generally, assessment of achievement was conducted by the 'Healthy Schools Award Co-ordinator' or teacher adviser. Ofsted Inspectors, or another external agent, were rarely used. The significant growth in Healthy Schools Awards in recent years is reinforced by the findings of a repeat survey undertaken in 1997 (BRMB, 1997). This showed that the proportion of units involved with an Award had risen to 69 per cent. Issues raised had changed little in the intervening

Table 7.3 Key statements from the Wessex Healthy Schools Award

Key statement	Description
A Comprehensive, co-ordinated curriculum and policies	The school should be working towards the National Curriculum Guidance Document no. 5 (Health Education). Its policies and programmes should be co-ordinated, comprehensive and progressive, and be reflected in the school development plan
B Wider community	Policies should reflect the school as part of the wider community.
C Smoke-free environment	The school should be working towards a smoke-free environment.
D Nutrition	Pupils should be educated and encouraged to make healthy food choices.
E Physical activity	The school should offer a wide range of physical activities which are accessible to all and in which working towards health becomes an important cultural practice within the school (National Curriculum Physical Education Statutory Orders).
F Responsibility for health	Schools should encourage young people to take responsibility for their own health.
G Staff health	The school should be a health-promoting workplace for staff.
H Environment	The school should promote a generally stimulating, clean, safe and tidy environment.
I Equal opportunities	There should be equal opportunity and access to health education for all who teach, learn and work in the school.

period; concerns over resources, and evaluation were expressed, with a keen desire to see more co-ordination and networking between schemes to ensure usage of common standards, and for exchange of good practice.

The Wessex Healthy Schools Award has also been evaluated in a three year controlled trial to assess its effectiveness on changing aspects of the organisation and environment of the school and on the health attitudes and behaviours of pupils. The study compared eleven intervention schools who undertook the award in the usual way, with five matched controls who had not applied to do the award. A range of both quantitative and qualitative measures were used to assess the impact of the award. An audit tool was developed as part of this project in order to assess the state of health education as an intrinsic element in secondary schools and to be able to quantitatively measure the degree of change in items during the period of the scheme (Moon *et al.*, 1997a). The tool is linked closely to the nine criteria for the award. Questions were formulated to explore each of these key areas in ways which reflect an holistic approach to becoming health-promoting schools. They were weighted, valued and scored by a team of health promotion specialists. Piloting demonstrated that the tool was acceptable if left for three senior staff (typically the headteacher and co-ordinators of physical and health education) to complete prior to a visit from the researcher who conducted a group discussion and collated agreed scores on a master copy.

The audit tool has proved successful as a diagnostic tool, and although it is detailed and requires commitment to complete it, it has stimulated assessment of health needs in schools and clearly identified areas for improvement. Staff have welcomed it, as have advisory teachers and others currently involved in school assessments, as it gives them a tangible and explicit record of achievement and progress. It will be used alongside other measures to evaluate the effect of the award process. It is hoped that it will be available for routine use as part of the future Healthy Schools Award scheme.

The Wessex Healthy Schools Award is an excellent example of a quality initiative in a health-promoting setting. Once again the development of the scheme demonstrated clear commitment to ensuring that the standards enshrined within it arose from and were agreed by a wide constituency of professional and user views. The lengthy period of piloting in the first group of schools ensured that the processes were acceptable to schools and could be accommodated within their busy timetables. However, as with the other schemes, with hindsight it is clear that the main target group, i.e. children, were not involved in the development process, thus the 'consumer' dimension is lacking. However the associated evaluation project is enabling assessment of the views of pupils through focus groups; and other non-teaching staff such as caretakers and caterers, and parents and governors through structured interviews (Moon *et al.*, 1997b) which will inform further revision of the scheme. The quality assurance processes combine elements of both CQI and ESI approaches. Whilst standards have been set externally to the individual schools involved thus ensuring comparability of achievement between schools, the selection of particular areas to work on, and the possibility of continuing this process over subsequent years addressing new areas, allows for continuous improvement in health promotion standards. Also the nature of the work towards each key statement is planned flexibly by each school according to their own needs. Quality initiatives such as this with externally derived standards do however require a strategy for regular review and updating of the standards. Since the Wessex Healthy Schools Award was developed the issues of substance misuse and bullying, for example, have become more important for schools and need formal recognition in the key statements in future revisions.

THE HEALTHY LEISURE AWARD

The last quality initiative to be considered is the Healthy Leisure Award which was developed by the Wessex Institute during 1995 and 1996. This followed on from the success of the schools award and the increasing interest expressed by leisure centres in health promotion. The development process was similar to that described for other schemes. A steering group with representation from health promotion, leisure management, primary care and local authorities met monthly initially to agree the key statements and performance indicators that would set the standards for a health-promoting leisure service. Having agreed these, seven pilot leisure centres, ranging from large local authority services to smaller private health clubs, were invited to work with the statements and provide feedback to the steering group to enable them to review and revise the documentation.

At this time many centres were already involved with local health promotion units to access various support services: staff training on courses such as 'Look After Yourself' and 'Helping People Change'; resources for national campaigns; and advice on setting up and running 'exercise prescription schemes' with local primary care teams. After eighteen months of development, the scheme was launched in the local health service region, and attracted a great deal of interest. In particular the professional body for this sector, the Institute of Leisure and Amenity Management (ILAM), recognised its potential for quality assurance in leisure services and became a partner in the scheme leading to a national launch in December 1996. ILAM markets the scheme to its members, the Wessex Institute provides training and monitoring to ensure quality, and an external training organisation undertakes the validations for centres (Rogers, 1997).

A year on over thirty centres have either achieved the Award or have applied to register for the scheme. In some instances local authorities who contract out for leisure services have included registration as a requirement in their tendering process. The registration fee includes a day's orientation and training for the centre co-ordinator and their local health promotion supporter. They have twelve months to complete and have to provide evidence of achievement of standards for all eight key statements in the areas of: community, environment; smoking policy; healthy food choices; range of activities; healthy workplace; training and exercise prescription scheme (see Table 7.4). This scheme followed the pattern of the others in ensuring through thorough consultation and testing, that the standards and quality assurance processes were acceptable and applicable to the setting concerned. Again, it was derived using a wide range of professional and management views, but lacked incorporation of the consumer perspective formally in planning. It conforms most closely to the ESI model, and of all the schemes it is perhaps the most rigorous, requiring achievement of minimum standards across all areas covered.

LESSONS LEARNT

This period of exploration of quality assurance principles in health promotion and evolution of processes to apply them has led to profound changes in the practice of health promoters in the UK. The quality 'culture' has taken root in practice and has led to a range of initiatives that both meet funders' needs for

Table 7.4 Key statements from the Healthy Leisure Award

Key statement	Description
A Community	Demonstrating that it is working as part of the community and with a range of organisations to promote healthy living.
B Environment	Promoting a generally stimulating, clean, safe and tidy environment.
C Smoking policy	Working towards a smoke-free environment by taking action on smoking issues.
D Healthy food choices	Encouraging users to make healthy food choices.
E Range of activities	Offering a wide range of activities which should be accessible to all with equity in provision and access.
F Healthy workplace	Providing a health promoting workplace for staff.
G Training	Providing appropriate training for staff.
H Exercise prescription scheme	Ensuring that where exercise prescription schemes are offered to local general practitioners, the centre provides a safe and effective programme.

accountability, and practitioners' needs for reflection and improvement of health promotion activities. The principles of 'user' involvement in derivation of quality assurance standards and processes has clearly been successful, and there is evidence of ownership and continued growth of quality improvements. However, the definition of users has not been clear. Whilst all the schemes described have balanced the needs of stakeholders, be they purchasers or providers of health promotion or the many others involved in delivery of interventions, it is evident that despite the rhetoric in health promotion of community participation in planning, this has yet to be fully achieved. The perspectives of the end-users of interventions, that is, those to whom the activity is directed, and whose health improvement is the goal, have not been adequately explored in most initiatives. In these settings-based approaches the views of school children, hospital patients and their families, and leisure centre users for example, need to be more fully integrated into the process. Where materials were assessed on consumers, such as in the evaluation indicators for alliances, they provided valuable insights and concerns that led to significant changes in the content. The familiar problems of time and resources are obviously a constraint in programme development, but the fact remains that when faced with the complexity of involving the diversity of users in health promotion programmes, too often we rely on the proxy perspective of the workers in contact with the consumer, rather than the consumer themselves.

The timing of the development of these approaches preceded or ran alongside the rising interest in evidence-based practice. Systematic reviews of the effectiveness of health promotion have been available only for the last year or so, and therefore it is not surprising that the standards incorporated in these quality assurance programmes and quality initiatives have generally been derived from professional knowledge of good practice, rather than based on research evidence. Whilst professional opinion draws upon this evidence, it is time to review the standards and criteria in the new context to integrate this emerging evidence into quality programmes. At the same time there is concern about the quality of health promotion interventions that are evaluated in research studies, and there are calls to include criteria for the quality of interventions in the inclusion criteria for reviews, and to give these equal emphasis to that required of the research methodology (Kok *et al.*, 1997; Speller and Webb, 1997).

Quality assurance in health promotion, based on the dimensions of professional, management and consumer quality, is an important aspect of the development of implementable interventions to ensure that they are acceptable and applicable to the setting, and based on current best evidence. Only such quality assured programmes should be subjected to the rigour and expense of effectiveness testing. If then proven effective they should be widely disseminated to practitioners with clear guidance on methods and standards expected, which would then be amenable to audit to ensure performance is maintained. Thus quality assurance and effectiveness research in health promotion are not separate endeavours, but are part of a cycle that would ensure quality in health promotion (Speller, 1998). Our work on the evaluation of the healthy schools award has managed to combine both aspects, but such examples are all too rare in health promotion research. The wide adoption of the healthy schools award approach, prior to its effect assessment, demonstrates clearly the way, as practitioners, we adopt good ideas with enthusiasm before they are adequately tested. It also shows the length of time and resources required to develop, implement and research large scale complex health promotion interventions; unfortunately the vision and commitment to extensive programmes of this nature is sadly lacking, despite calls from all the effectiveness reviews to undertake more research on UK practice in health promotion.

The experience we have to date has shown the enthusiasm of practitioners for quality assurance, and the appeal of quality assured interventions which appears to improve their uptake and adoption in the wider community. It also demonstrates the need to involve a range of users, including more representatives of consumers in the derivation of standards, and to balance the application of explicit external standards with processes that allow for entry at different points, tailoring to local circumstance and room for continuous growth and improvement. Based on the experience of these and similar programmes, and with the incorporation of evidence of effectiveness, the next logical step is for the agreement of national standards and quality frameworks, endorsed either by national health promotion agencies or government bodies, to ensure effective health promotion practice.

References

BRMB International (1997) *Health Promoting Schools National Survey Report, May 1997.* London: BRMB.

Department of Health (1989) *Working for Patients.* London: HMSO.

Department of Health (1991) *NHS Research and Development Strategy* – Guidance for Regions. September 1991. London: DOH.

Department of Health (1992) *The Health of the Nation: A Strategy for Health in England.* London: HMSO.

Department of Health (1994) *Health Promoting Hospitals*, 1128, September 1994. London: DOH.

Duffy, S. (1997) *Partnerships in Action: Working towards a Smoke-free Scotland.* Edinburgh: Health Education Board for Scotland.

Evans, D., Head, M. J. and Speller, V. (1994) *Assuring Quality in Health Promotion. How to Develop Standards of Good Practice.* London: Health Education Authority.

Funnell, R., Oldfield, K. and Speller, V. (1995) *Towards Healthier Alliances. A tool for Planning, Evaluating and Developing Healthy Alliances.* London: Health Education Authority.

Joss, R. and Kogan, M. (1995) *Advancing Quality: Total Quality Management in the NHS.* Birmingham: Oxford University Press.

Kok, G., van den Borne, B. and Mullen, P.D. (1997) Effectiveness of health education and health promotion: meta-analyses of effect studies and determinants of effectiveness. *Patient Education and Counselling* 30, 19–27.

Moon, A. M., Rogers, E., Mullee, M.A., Speller, V. and Roderick, P.J. (1997a) The Wessex Healthy Schools Award (WHSA) evaluation – developing an audit tool for schools. *The Canadian Journal of Cardiology* 13, Supplement B, 126B.

Moon, A. M., Rogers, E., Mullee, M.A., Speller, V. and Roderick, P.J. (1997b) Wessex Healthy Schools Award (WHSA) evaluation – the perceptions of school staff. *The Canadian Journal of Cardiology*, 13, Supplement B, 127B.T.

Ovretveit, J. (1992) *Health Service Quality.* Oxford: Blackwell Scientific.

Ovretveit, J. (1996) Quality in health promotion. *Health Promotion International* 11(1), 55–62.

Rogers, E. (1997) *The Healthy Leisure Award Portfolio.* University of Southampton: Wessex Institute for Health Research and Development.

Rogers, E., Taylor, P. and Gott, D. (1993) *The Wessex Healthy Schools Award.* Winchester: Wessex Institute for Public Health Medicine.

Rogers, E., Moon, A.M., Mullee, M.A., Speller, V. and Roderick, P.J. (1998) Developing the 'health-promoting school': a national survey of healthy schools awards. *Public Health* 112, 37–40.

Royle, J. and Speller, V. (1996) Assuring quality in health promotion. Paper presented at Quality Assessment in Health Promotion and Education: the 3rd European Conference on Effectiveness, Turin, Italy, September 1996.

Rushmere, A. (1997) *Health-promoting Hospitals: Audit and Accreditation Process for Organisational Development.* University of Southampton: Wessex Institute for Health Research and Development.

Speller, V. (1998) Quality assurance programmes: their development and contribution to improving effectiveness in health promotion. In Weston, R. and Scott, D. (eds) *Evaluating Health Promotion.* Cheltenham: Stanley Thornes.

Speller, V. and Webb, D. (1997) Looking at the quality of health promotion interventions in the systematic review process: redressing the balance. In *Reviews of Effectiveness: Their Contribution to Evidence Based Practice and Purchasing in Health Promotion. Workshop Report, 19th Mar. 1997.* London: Health Education Authority.

Speller, V., Evans, D. and Head M.J. (1997) Developing quality assurance standards for health promotion practice in the U.K. *Health Promotion International* 12(3), 215–224.

Part III

Approaches to synergism

Chapter 8

Paradigms, values and quality criteria in health promotion: an application to primary health care

Alain Deccache and Jean Laperche

INTRODUCTION

This chapter addresses the links between health promotion ideology and practice and different aspects of evaluation of effectiveness and quality. It reminds us that health promotion is based upon a specific ideology and values which imply certain conceptual frameworks and models. It also tries to demonstrate why and how methods and criteria for practice and evaluation need to be coherent and complementary with health promotion concepts and their assumptions.

It presents the professional, scientific and ethical basis of such options, and their practical implications. It finally tries to answer the questions: What kind of criteria should the evaluation of quality in health promotion take into account, and how can it be done?

The chapter will consist of two sections. The first is a brief presentation and discussion of health promotion concepts, evaluation and quality, and of their implications for practice. The second section applies this discussion to a health promotion project, on which the authors have been working since 1994: the development of quality health promotion practice in thirty primary health care centres, focusing on patient and community participation.

HEALTH PROMOTION CONCEPTS AND THEIR LINK WITH EVALUATION METHODOLOGIES

In a slight adaptation of the Ottawa Charter's approach, Tones (1992) defines health promotion simply as 'the product of actions of health education and of healthy public policy'. This implies that health promotion, either at a legal, environmental, social or health level, cannot be conceived without a simultaneous health education and health policy.

COMMUNITY PARTICIPATION: NEW ROLES FOR THE POPULATION AND THE PROFESSIONALS

Health promotion fits in with a particular ideological movement: community participation. This movement sees the individual or the community as active decision-makers, as citizens and not only as health consumers. Their views can be identical to those of health and social institutions, or on the contrary, and sometimes alternately, in conflict with these institutions. The same applies for the health promoter, who is first of all an agent of change and of empowerment. Depending on the situation, health promoters are at the service of the community and its health, and sometimes at the service of a health policy or institution. This dichotomy appears through different existing organisations: from state agencies to non-governmental organisations (NGOs), patients or health users associations, for example, and reflects varied, and sometimes opposing views and approaches to health promotion (Caplan and Holland, 1990; Taylor, 1990). Thus, it leads to different processes and methods of action, of needs assessment, of 'implication' of various actors involved (i.e. decision-makers, professionals, researchers, industries). For example, health needs and health promotion needs are not only defined by experts on the basis of theoretical models of health determinants and epidemiological data. They also have to be defined by the community itself, which has to put its priorities in balance with those of experts.

AN INTERDISCIPLINARY APPROACH AND VIEWPOINTS

Developed from a basis in public health and various social sciences, health promotion and education are based upon different paradigms, from epidemiology to psychology and anthropology. Several authors (Liedekerke *et al.*, 1990; Briziarelli, 1989; Tones, 1992; Bury, 1988) have warned against an exclusive use of disciplines of public health to understand, act, plan and evaluate in health promotion.

For example, in health promotion, the concept of health itself is double sided. It is an epidemiological, objective and measurable state, but it may also be considered as a subjective, individual and social state. In practice this implies the integration of actions aimed at the prevention of disease and those aimed at the maintenance and improvement of health. Thus it has two objects of interest: health and disease (or risk). It also suggests a combination of the usual vertical approach (by pathology, themes or risks) with a transverse or horizontal approach (by public or situation). Finally, it widens the health perspective, from a (narrow) problem solving process, in which needs are defined on the basis of deficiencies, risks, negative aspects, to life projects and expectations of social groups and individuals, i.e. the positive aspects of their life and health.

It leads to 'pro-action' as a complement to 're-action', which is the basis of the classical prevention process.

IMPLICATIONS FOR EVALUATION

Corresponding to ideological choices in health promotion, there are theoretical options, a certain view of evaluation and quality concepts and therefore methods and techniques that can differ from those used in most cases so far. For a long time, in evaluation, the public health approach has prevailed. In this context, evaluation is conceived as the measurement of effectiveness (mainly epidemiological). This does not answer the questions 'how or why does it work?' or 'what can be improved?' In other approaches, such as educational sciences, evaluation is considered as 'a collection of information aimed at decision-making'. The evaluation of effectiveness is part of this approach, together with the evaluation of process, needs, impact, etc. Sometimes, the social marketing and communication approach is used, with its market surveys, audience segmentation, readability, penetration or effectiveness evaluations, etc. More and more, the anthropological approach and its methods, including ethnography, has come to reinforce the previous approaches.

Educational sciences brought to a restrictive definition of the process, such as 'throughput', the larger meaning of 'all the things that occur', including input and throughput (de Ketele and Renders, 1986). This implies that methods and processes of needs analysis, of objectives and priorities setting, as well as the implementation of health promotion projects, should be the purposes of quality assessment. Even the modes of action and interaction between actors are taken into account and lead to the evaluation of ethical and ideological aspects of projects. Another example concerns the evaluation of effects. Green (1986) distinguishes two kinds of effects: impact and results. Impact includes direct and indirect intermediate effects, targeted or not. In health education, any change of knowledge, social representations, perceptions and attitudes, can be considered as the impact. The results are 'final' effects often in the mid or long term, in terms of morbidity, mortality, access to services or care and health costs. Evaluating effectiveness is about checking whether, and to what extent, targeted objectives were effectively met. Evaluating quality is assessing the ability of the implementation process (strategy, means, procedures, interactions etc) to produce the desired effects.

QUALITY ASSURANCE IN HEALTH PROMOTION

Quality assurance is 'a systematic process by which desirable levels of quality are described, the degree of feasibility of these levels is defined, and improvement decisions are taken and implemented' (Wright et al., 1992). Quality is defined as 'all the elements and characteristics of a service which determine its ability to fulfill the needs of a public' (BSI, 1978). Therefore, assessing the quality of health promotion and education means implementing a programme of quality assurance, identifying key components of this programme, setting quality standards and evaluation criteria, assessing the performance of activities, taking improvement decisions and ensuring a follow-up of these decisions.

Now, in quality assurance, there are two distinct approaches. The first one, called 'external standards inspection' or ESI consists in establishing criteria of quality, evaluating them and improving them. The second one, called 'continuous quality improvement' or CQI considers the activity or service as a process and views quality assessment as part of the process, involving all the participants, professionals and users themselves (Ovretveit, 1994).

In the field of health/disease and care, the quality concept was brought in as part of a need to control health costs. In this perspective, quality assurance is an objectivist process, using mainly quantitative methods and considering subjective aspects (patients' views, for example) only through objective and predefined criteria. In this respect, the ESI approach is still mainly used.

The CQI approach is much more relevant within the context of health promotion. Because it puts every participant in the process in an active position, and because it is a participative process, it fits better in the health promotion ideology. Lastly, it rejects predefined evaluation and allows the creation of new criteria and indicators for the evaluation and the measurement of processes and effects, rather than only using the existing epidemiological, biomedical ones. Therefore, there are clearly several standpoints and paradigms which complement one another, and offer various ways of assessing quality.

APPROPRIATE OBJECTS, METHODS AND CRITERIA FOR QUALITY ASSESSMENT

To assess quality, it is necessary to understand how a process can result in certain effects. As in any form of evaluation, criteria are necessary. These criteria have to be appropriate to the objects under evaluation, that is, to the process specific to every action or programme.

Only then, does it become possible to define 'good practice standards', on the basis of clear and relevant criteria. Now the selection of criteria is not neutral. It is determined by the conceptual framework that sets up the kind of appropriate practice. In order to break this figure of eight, Evans *et al.* (1994) have empirically described several 'good practice criteria' for the six functions of the health promotion work (planning, project management, evaluation, training, professional information, methodological counselling). Some of these criteria are: an explicit and shared philosophy of project, a clear definition of health decisions based on needs analyses, real intersectorial collaboration, active participation and involvement of the population, reflection and self-evaluation of the process, etc.

These fundamental elements of health promotion can be grouped in general and inevitable categories of criteria:

- criteria related to the programme, i.e. to all planned activities: their types, implementation, components, adequacy to needs (and not only to problems) expressed or not;
- criteria concerning agents and contributors: their skills, interactions, abilities to encourage the emergence of the community needs and to support actions;
- criteria related to the involved community, public or individuals: quality of participants, their level of participation, satisfaction, etc.;
- criteria of management of available resources and constraints;
- criteria of interaction
  - between parts of a programme,
  - between different involved programmes and systems (i.e. inter-sectoriality, the respective parts of health education and social policy),
  - complementarity of vertical (by theme or risk) and transverse (by public or situation) approaches;
- criteria related to theoretical choices, to underlying values, such as acceptability, equity, accessibility, ethical aspects, and to the relevance of methods and techniques to effective philosophical and conceptual choices. The difference between participation, activism and manipulation is sometimes subtle. Limits between the health of the public and public health are not well defined. The individual's interest and the collectivity's interest are often conflictual.

Between 'scientific complexity' and 'political necessity' the position of 'social relevance' in health promotion needs to be maintained. Among the different types of possible criteria, choices have to be made according to specific situations. Between 'historical' criteria, based on experience, 'normative' criteria, based on pilot group consensus, and 'absolute' criteria, based on the ideal situation (Green, 1986), there are also 'negotiated' criteria which combines all the others.

These proposals put quality assessment in health promotion and education half-way between 'external standards inspection' (ESI) and 'continuous quality improvement' (CQI). An alternative more in accordance with the principles of health promotion and education would consist in defining general criteria of quality, or categories of criteria, operationalised by specific indicators, defined by the actors of the considered system or programme. It would acknowledge the importance of certain qualitative characteristics, such as well-being, meeting expectations, community and social relevance, etc. These elements are not often measurable but they are needed to help us ensure we take all the aspects of processes and effects of health promotion into consideration.

Lastly, the remaining question is how to put these reflections and choices into practice, and how to build and implement a quality assurance process which would fulfil the following conditions: be participative and 'community centred', to ensure an interdisciplinary integration (of subjective and objective health, of disease prevention and health maintenance, of vertical and transverse approaches, of problem based and situation based work), have a wide vision of the process (including needs assessment, priority setting, action planning, etc.), and focus on both impact and results, and to address ethical questions. The answer lies partly in the way quality criteria are defined. The second section of this chapter will focus on practical aspects of this process and show how it can be started in health settings where care and prevention are being linked to health promotion work.

AN APPLICATION TO A HEALTH PROMOTION PROJECT IN PRIMARY HEALTH CARE

The following case study presents the process of implementation of quality assurance, in a project in which primary care centres try to integrate curative, preventive and health promotion work within a community participation approach. Difficulties and achievements are presented and discussed.

Context of the project

The Belgian health system is built up around private and public hospitals and general and specialized private practice. However, an alternative sub-system was created in 1975: about a hundred general practice, primary health care centres in which multidisciplinary teams put together all categories of health care professionals in a private practice oriented towards primary health care. These centres called 'Maisons médicales' are grouped within a federation, the FMMCSF (Fédération des Maisons Médicales et Collectifs de Santé Francophones). Besides the fact they opted for a social and comprehensive type of medicine that leads them to curative and preventive care, these 'maisons médicales' share a common health philosophy described in a 'Charte des Maisons Médicales'. This charter gives a central position to health users and their autonomy, to community health, to non-medical determinants of health and to partnership with local social and political networks. Its project is based on values of equity, quality of care, efficiency, autonomy and social solidarity.

Besides the usual system of payment on service, one-third of the 'maisons médicales' was authorised by the Ministry of Health to get paid a fixed rate established on the basis of the number of patients registered to each participating 'maison médicale'. This funding method facilitates a preventive, multidisciplinary and social medical practice.

In 1992 and 1993, the FMMCSF undertook a large survey, carried out by the Université Libre de Bruxelles PROMES team, over 1,200 patients and 278 health care professionals. The study focused on common features and differences between expectations and representations in terms of care and prevention (Levêque and Roubaix, 1993; Laperche and Delpierre, 1994).

In order to improve the proposed prevention services and to develop health promotion practices in its 'maisons médicales', the FMMCSF organised a large pilot action research project. The project was funded by the Ministry of Health. Between 1994 and 1996, the project 'Acting together in prevention' was joined by 23 teams (Gosselain and Laperche, 1996). The project started with a review of actual prevention practices within the participating centres, an information collection stage on activities and projects, training on project management, evaluation and communication at the request of participating teams, and methodological counselling by promoters and researchers of the FMMCSF. In order to respect the teams' autonomy and the values of the charter, priorities and objectives were defined by each team itself. The Federation offered support in organisational analysis and effectiveness evaluation, methods for the involvement of patients in projects and decisions, co-ordination within and among teams, appropriate methods of definition of objectives, planning, improvement of effectiveness of actions, intersectoriality and collaboration with social and health organisations and networks, dealing with obstacles inside or outside projects, funding projects, etc.

A first intermediate evaluation was carried out in late 1995 (Miermans, 1995). Amongst the conclusions, it emphasised the following needs. Out of 27 action themes or subjects listed in 1995 (the total was 55 identified actions), 6 used a global approach and were oriented towards health and not merely disease prevention. Subjects were: family planning, food, physical activity, group meetings on health, self-help groups, children's playgrounds and safety in the neighbourhood. Each project involved helping patients, clients and their families in getting easier access to services, organising health information and education, participating in actions and obtaining support from local authorities. But most of the projects were still prevention oriented (immunisation and screening programmes mainly), and they lacked a systematic approach and real equal access to everyone concerned.

Many projects were organised in an intersectoral way, in collaboration with other social, health or educational organisations. However, the patient-users' position was limited even when they were asked to collaborate. They were not involved very much in priority setting, decision, choice and in the conception of prevention and health promotion and education activities. The promotion of users' real participation as an important aim of the project had to be reinforced.

The relevance of many projects was considered through their medical aspects (health needs) and oriented towards medical actions (immunisations, screenings, check-ups). In these projects, health communication and education were only seen as a means to reinforce the population coverage. However, most of them were also socially oriented and relevant. The prevention process, considered as the 'health' side of the care system, was considered insufficient to improve the quality and implementation of the institution's values (autonomy, equity, effectiveness, etc.). It seemed necessary to widen it to health promotion.

DEFINING QUALITY AND CHOOSING CRITERIA

Since 1996, the project has been redirected towards the development of quality assurance and health promotion. Thirty teams take part in this project and
are encouraged to widen their view and their practices and to make them
systematically more adequate in terms of quality criteria. The total number of
local projects reached 100. Several general meetings have been organised for
the participating teams and their representatives, in order to redefine health
promotion and its implications in primary health care, along with an introduction to the quality assurance process.

As a guide to practice and evaluation, the project's promoters and reseachers
decided to use two sources of recommendations. The first comes from general
practice – primary health care (Donabedian, 1988; Hutchinson, 1993; Grol,
1990), and is based mainly on the model of external standards inspection
(ESI) and evaluation by medico-epidemiological methods. The second source
is recommendations from health promotion (Evans *et al.*, 1994; Ovretveit,
1996; Macdonald, 1996), which favour the model of continuous quality
improvement (CQI) and participative and qualitative evaluation. Usual theoretical
referents of general practice appear to be partly in conflict with those of health
promotion and of the Federation's institutional values. These values vary (from
efficiency to equity and participation), but methods of action and evaluation
available only allow such effects as coverage, morbidity or cost-effectiveness.
Even users' satisfaction is considered in medical standards as an 'external' and
predefined object.

Confronted with the risk of an evaluation incoherent with the initial objectives
and values of the project, the situation seems to be paradoxical: how to reconcile
a quality assessment that respects the usual scientific referents with social relevance
and the positive health orientation of the project? Can primary health care
teams accept imposed external criteria to improve their practices and at the
same time be participative and respectful of patients' and users' choices? How
can the clients' autonomy be reinforced without retaining sufficient professional
autonomy?

In order to integrate the two reference models and the project's values, the
promoters made two choices. The first concerns the selection of quality criteria.
A selection of twenty available criteria was submitted to participating teams.
Thirteen criteria (Table 8.1) were chosen and agreed upon during meetings in
which they were presented, discussed and submitted to the participating teams'
approval. They are used as much for evaluation as for the definition of objectives
and priorities to improve the quality of actions.

The second choice concerns the definition of quality indicators and of evaluation
methods to be used. Although indicators already exist, a participative evaluation
requires them to be negotiated with participants. Besides, they should be relevant
to practices which differ from one team to another. A qualitative process was
chosen. It consisted of sorting out, from information and data brought by

Table 8.1 Quality criteria and consensual definitions

Quality factors	Definition
Relevance	The process or strategy is *relevant* when it aims at answering identified needs, whether they are medical, social, individual, institutional or related to the project's values. Needs may be defined objectively or subjectively, by health care professionals or users, quantitatively or qualitatively.
Efficacy	It defines a process or strategy which is built upon information or processes of which the efficacy was already proven in specific conditions. It can be medical (medical consensus), methodological (recommended method or means), epidemiological (coverage rate) etc.
Effectiveness	The process or strategy is *effective* when it meets its objectives, that is, if positive effects are those that had been targeted, in the specific context of action. It can be defined in one or several terms: biomedical (morbidity-mortality), psychosocial (attitudes, health representations ...), behavioural, communicative (reached public, level of retention ...), organisational (collaboration network, co-ordination ...).
Efficiency	The process or strategy is *efficient* when it can give the best effects with the lowest costs, or with the best use of existing resources. It can be financial, procedural, organisational.
Globality	The process or strategy is *global* when it is concerned explicitly and simultaneously with different aspects of a person, a patient or a community: biomedical, health, psychosocial, social, environmental, legal and educational aspects.
Continuity	The process or strategy is *continuous* when it ensures an appropriate counselling in time, of the project or the patient, by the same concerned persons. It implies more than a follow-up, which does not require the permanence of professionals, and can be assured by different health care providers.
Integration	The process or strategy is *integrated* when it makes sure that concerns for disease and complication prevention, health education and promotion are *included* in other (daily or usual) activities.
Equity and accessibility	The process or strategy is *equitable* (and accessible) when it concerns and aims at reaching all people, or those who need it most, such as deprived or disadvantaged people.
User's participation and autonomy	The process or strategy is *participative* when it allows patients to take part in care, when it helps them to express their choices and needs, and to fulfil them. Such a process implies a sharing of decision-making, a consideration of the patient's view and of social, personal and family acceptability besides health and medical acceptability.
Subsidiarity	It defines the process or strategy which acknowledges the roles and positions of various concerned organisations and contributors, and which encourages a sharing of roles and tasks according to existing skills and services. It aims at facilitating the access to services, using actual competences and missions and at avoiding misuse of health promotion services.
Systematisation	The process or strategy is *systematic* when it aims at reaching *all* concerned persons and patients.

Table 8.1 continued

Quality factors	Definition
Satisfaction of health care team and/or users	The process or strategy is *satisfying* (for providers and/or the community) when it meets *expectations and wishes* (expressed needs) of participants. It concerns services, as much as procedures and relationships, costs and effects.
Collectivity Interdisciplinarity and team work	The process or strategy is *collective* and interdisciplinary when it associates all the providers and the team's professionals in planned actions. It implies a broad and integrative view of concerned health disciplines and social work.

Source: Deccache *et al.* (1997b).

participants, elements indicating their views and ways of evaluating quality. Therefore, relevant indicators have been inferred from observations, but most of them still meet technical expert recommendations.

The purposes of evaluation were: to assess the quality of methodological counselling offered by the Federation to the 'maisons médicales'; to ensure that current projects are in accordance with criteria of quality; to describe changes which would have occurred in practice from the beginning of the project, in quantity (number of projects) as well as quality (meeting quality criteria); to describe effective changes, as a result of an expected rebound effect, in practices other than those related to health promotion (curative practices, accommodation, organisational and care relationship practices); to prepare adjustments and follow-up (supervision and evaluation) of developed projects and of changes in practice.

The last two objectives are still under evaluation.

Four of the nine methods of evaluation identified by WONCA (Roland and Jamoulle, 1995), were used together here: audit (data collection on practices, discussion and proposals), search for a consensus (critical discussion on institutional or scientific directives), peer review and external experts' advice. The evaluation process had to be participative, and thus coherent with the philosophy of the project. To guarantee this, four principles are respected. (1) Criteria of quality are determined in common by the FMMCSF (on the basis of its charter and on international recommendations of quality in primary health care and in health promotion) and by participating teams. (2) The analyses of collected data are redirected to teams for feedback, additional information and reaction. (3) Among the common criteria, 'local' relevance for the development and follow-up of each team is discussed, and each team selects the criteria on which it intends to improve its practice. (4) Evaluation is made internally within teams, and externally by project promoters and external evaluators.

The information collected is qualitative (estimations, observations, analyses of documents and interviews) and quantitative (health data, results of surveys, immunisation rates collected by participating centres). It is collected by promoters from three sources: existing reports, documents and compilation of project descriptions (promoters analysed them using the list of selected criteria of quality and indicators); observations and teams' group interviews, carried out in 1997; and additional information and feedback brought by participating teams after the first analysis. These data allowed assessment of the situation after the first two years, and at the beginning of the quality assurance stage. It was also useful in preparing follow-up to developed projects and to changes that have been implemented as part of the quality assurance process.

Building appropriate indicators

The most participative stage of the evaluation is the common construction of quality indicators and items for evaluation (Deccache *et al.*, 1997a, 1997b). A double analysis was carried out: an 'intra-team', where all the information collected for each team was synthesised, and an 'inter-team', where all the syntheses were put together and compared. Then it was possible to spot the indicators each team favours and to create 'scales' that turned criteria of quality into indicators. For example, 'patients' participation' was interpreted in different ways by the teams: as the systematic information of patients about planned prevention activities, as a regular data collection of patients' advice and expectations and their satisfaction during the projects, as a systematic involvement of patients (or their representatives) in the design and implementation of projects, etc. This information allowed the development of a 'patients' participation' continuance, on which a team or a project could evolve, from a narrow vision (to inform patients) to a larger vision (to ensure that they take part in decisions and projects), more in accordance with the concept of participation.

This is an example of the 'patients' participation' criterion.

Minimum				Maximum
to inform patients	to listen	to collect expectations	to consult on projects/services	to actively involve

The 'relevance' criterion is another example of the fact that a factor can take unexpected forms and still be meaningful to the actors. For this criterion, indicators of relevance vary between medical relevance (related to health status), social relevance (related to employment issues affecting health), environmental relevance (related to housing salubrity), individual relevance (related to patients' demands), organisational relevance (related to the team's common project) or values-oriented relevance (to encourage participation). The 'health' concern remains present whatever the kind of relevance.

From one criterion to another, modalities vary. For 'participation', it is a scale with ranked categories. For 'relevance', the modality is unranked categories, where the result may be a sum of several indicators. For some criteria, several indicators appear in parallel, depending on the kind of objective, but none of them prevails. For 'effectiveness', if the aim is health education, the indicator is 'the reachability level of the targeted public' or 'the knowledge level of the population' or the 'behaviour change'. If the aim is 'to vaccinate concerned people', the indicator will be 'the immunisation coverage rate' or 'the re-immunisation rate'. If the aim is 'a better accessibility', the indicator is 'rate or number of new immunisations' or even 'characteristics of recently reached users'.

If the relevance and reliability of data seem to have been more favoured than validity, it all depends on the nature of the information collected. Medical or cognitive data are measurable and can be validated. Others are qualitative and only make sense according to the people who give them. One could quantify participation or accessibility, but the question is to know if it is relevant or appropriate. Finally, as the indicators and their modalities were rebuilt starting from information collected by the teams, it was possible to send them back (for feedback and correction) 'full scales' even where there were only one or two modalities in the beginning. In this way, the evaluation presents a formative aspect providing the teams with other possible indicators and modalities which they can decide to add to their own objectives.

The evaluation also emphasised several important practices and elements which otherwise would not have been revealed. 'Efficacy' is clearly defined only for medical preventive projects and from medical consensus. Many projects have no specific medical aspect. But as teams only refer to accepted knowledge in a certain field of prevention (the closest to classical medicine), several projects lacked references to efficacy, because of the absence of clear recommendations. This will orientate the project towards dissemination to teams of evidence-based practice in health education and community health.

'Effectiveness' is defined in many ways: on the scale, the minimum level is to have reached people belonging to the targeted public. 'Immunisation' projects assess their effectiveness by the immunisation coverage they reach (for which there are reference levels). Other elements, scarcely objectivised (or difficult to objectivise) appear, such as reaching a public that is difficult to reach (when trying to improve accessibility), measurement of patients' or teams' satisfaction, improvement of patients' quality of life, evolution of the patients' demand (in terms of autonomy and of decrease of useless demands of curative care), and evaluating the improvement of communication between patients and health care professionals and among health care professionals themselves.

'Efficiency' is scarcely addressed. Conceptual and methodological issues are indeed extremely important in this matter. The only concerned teams address efficiency in programmes where efficacy is obvious and where effectiveness is objectively measurable from data collected during the project (with no additional data collection as would be necessary when the evolution of well-being is assessed). Thus they try to address efficiency by comparing achieved coverage rates with different procedures, or by measuring the decrease of the demand of individual care and the increase of the demand of collective prevention (in a team financed on flat rate, this is indeed an element of efficiency).

'Globality' seems to be important and frequent. Almost all teams have prevention activities on several levels (medical, psychosocial, well-being). Moreover, globality is explained in a more specific way. In some teams, social issues are at the origin of the definition of the main target public and of objectives. In other teams, the focus is on the person's globality, and on the search for a balance between positive aspects of prevention and the risk of making people more dependent on the medical system.

Regarding 'integration', several indicators appear as well. The first one is the presence of curative and preventive activities in the same service. This first indicator is acknowledged by all teams. Some teams even consider that prevention is of utmost importance in their work. Another indicator consists in offering prevention services during a consultation, even if these services are not related to the aim of the consultation. The result of such a process has only been assessed for immunisation so far. It could easily be assessed in other situations (breast cancer screening, self-help groups, chronic disease compliance). The third indicator is to define, starting from the consultation, situations that could be better dealt with by prevention rather than by care. This concerns, for example, physical activity groups, obese women, cancer self-help groups. Health maintenance, without reference to potential or existing problems, is not yet very much developed, probably due to consultation reasons, patients' demands and health professionals' competences.

'Accessibility' and 'equity' are fundamental criteria for most of the maisons médicales. However, accessibility is most often addressed financially. It is assessed by the mode of payment (flat rate) or by free provision of care or even by delayed payment. Besides, several maisons médicales have developed projects aimed at certain categories of deprived patients (housing projects, health solidarity projects). Accessibility is also seen on a cultural level, with the research for health communication means adapted to a hardly educated public. Finally, it is sometimes seen on a practical level (attaching a vaccine prescription to a reminder letter). Some teams make the use of preventive services easier.

The concept of 'subsidiarity' is not used very often. It is mainly thought of as a result of the team's reflection about its roles and time or skills limits, about the interest of partnerships with existing organisations and networks, or about the patients' autonomy. 'Systematisation' consists in developing procedures in order to reach all concerned people and to realise all necessary actions. As far as the team is concerned, it means standardising strategies among the different health care providers. At the public level, it aims at reaching most of those targeted.

' Patient satisfaction' is often considered as one of the criteria of the effectiveness or relevance of a project. Therefore, it is a major criterion for the teams' work. Patient participation is seen as an indicator of their satisfaction. So is the fact that they start requesting of their own volition activities or services which have been proposed to them before, as in the case of immunisation.

'Interdisciplinarity and team work' are often considered as attained when a search for a consensus on procedures or at least on shared values is achieved. Besides an organisation which encourages communication (teams meetings, co-ordination tools), some teams have developed a transdisciplinary 'prevention' group, sometimes involving users and families.

Some lessons from this project

There are many quality criteria and some of them even cover two or more dimensions. In this project, we have focused on thirteen of them. Theoretically, it would have been necessary to evaluate or measure at least thirteen different 'dimensions' in order to assess quality. The process would have been much too complex. The project allowed every team to choose its own priorities and criteria, and therefore to decide what to measure. In the long run, all thirteen criteria will have been evaluated, but in a much more acceptable and affordable way. The choice of relevant indicators was also challenging. For each defined criterion, several indicators appeared to be useful. But among the participating teams, some have chosen certain indicators rather than others, because they seemed more relevant to them. Thus, for the sake of relevance, we had to accept that for the same criterion, different indicators would be used, and that comparison among centres would sometimes be impossible.

Lastly, it could have been easier to 'make measurements' using existing objective criteria, but it would have been contradictory and definitely inappropriate to the project. Besides, teams could not have adopted the process (made it theirs) and integrated it in their practices, which is the main aim of the project and of quality assurance. The aim of this project description was to show how the recommendations made in the first part of the chapter could be implemented.

Participation was reached through the evaluation process itself. By allowing participants to make their own choices, the project was coherent with its assumptions, and avoided the paradox of the 'do as I say, and not as I do'. It allows teams to improve their health promotion work, and develop real participative actions with the population concerned. The next step for the project is to monitor and follow up this transfer to patients and population. Only then we will know if this complex process was really sucessful, even if its first step is undoubtedly reached.

The quality criteria chosen included reference to subjective and objective health, to disease prevention and health maintenance, to vertical and transverse approaches, and to problem- and situation-based actions. Although these aspects are not yet always integrated in practice, they are now part of the process and should be reached in the future. Finally, efficacy as well as effectiveness will take into account impact and results, medical and non-medical effects, quantitative and qualitative changes, as was recommended. Ethics and coherence with the project's values are present in several criteria, from relevance to accessibility and autonomy.

The projects upon which this reflection is based are still in their early stages, or at least their interest to health promotion is. However, it already seems possible to ensure an operational coherence between theoretical choices, values and orientations of a project in health promotion and the methods and means used to evaluate and to assess the quality of such a project. Though it is apparently more complex and difficult to standardise, a participative and creative process of quality assurance is realistic and can result in the improvement of practices and their efficiency.

Note

The authors wish to thank Yves Gosselain, Marianne Prévost and Jacques Morel, from the FMMCSF, who are carrying out the project and its evaluation, and have provided most of the information used in this paper. Thanks too to the members of the supervision scientific team: Dr Cabut, Dr Duval, Mrs Miermans (Université de Liège), Dr Berghmans et Levêque (Université Libre de Bruxelles) and Dr Heremans (Université catholique de Louvain). The project is funded by the Belgian French Community Ministry of Health, Social Affairs and Health Promotion.

References

Briziarelli, L. (1989) Evaluation in health education, in Mahan C. and Tinarelli M. (eds) *Consultation on Evaluation on Health Education*. Perugia: Experimental Centre for Health Education, IUHE/EURO: 10–21.

BSI: British Standards Institution (1978) *British Standards Quality Vocabulary*. London: BS 4778.

Bury, J.A. (1988) Education pour la Santé; Concepts enjeux Planifications. De Boeck-Université, coll. Bruxelles. *Savoirs et santé*: 232.

Caplan, R. and Holland, R. (1990) Rethinking health education theory. *Health Education Journal*, 49, 1: 10–12.

Deccache, A., Prevost, M., Laperche, J. and Gosselain, Y. (1997a) Evaluation d'un Projet de Promotion de la Santé en Maison Médicale. Bruxelles: Rapport au Ministère de la santé, July (unpublished report).

Deccache, A., Prevost, M., Laperche, J., Gosselain, Y. and Morel, J. (1997b) *Evaluation du Projet Agir ensemble en Prevention, Rapport au Ministère de la Santé de la Communauté Française de Belgique*, Bruxelles: Fédération des Maisons Médicales, p. 77.

De Ketele, J.M. and Renders, X. (1986) Méthodologie du Recueil d'Informations, 1ère Edition, ed. De Boeck université, coll.Bruxelles. *Pédagogies en développement*: 198.

Donabedian, A. (1988) The quality of care: how can it be assessed? *Jama* 260, 1,743–1,748.

Evans, D., Head, M.J. and Speller, V. (1994) *Assuring Quality in Health Promotion: How to Develop Standards of Good Practice*. London: Health Education Authority, 106.

Gosselain, Y. and Laperche, J. (1996) Agir en Prévention, unpublished report, Brussels: Féderation des maisons médicales, 22.

Green, L.W. (1986) The theory of participation. *Advances in Health Education and Promotion* vol. 1, part A. Jai Press, 211–236.

Grol, R. (1990) National standard setting for quality of care in general practice: attitudes of general practitioners and response to a set of standards. *British Journal of General Practice* 40, 361–364.

Hutchinson, A. (1993) Primary care quality improvement. *Huisarts en Wetenschap* 36(13).

Jonkers, R. (1989) Effectiveness in health education, in Mahan, C. and Tinarelli, M. (eds) *Consultation on Evaluation of Health Education*, Perugia: Experimental Centre for Health Education, IUHE/EURO, 22–36.

Laperche, J. and Delpierre, V. (1994) La Prévention: Côté Soignants, Côté Patients, Brussels. *Education Santé* 88, 9–14.

Leveque, A. and de Roubaix, J. (1993) Education pour la Prévention, unpublished report, Brussels: Promes-ulb Ed.

Liedekerke *et al.* (1990) *Effectiveness of Health Education: Review and Analysis.* Dutch Health Education Centre, ed. Assen, The Netherlands: Van Gorcum/Uitgeverij voor Gezonheidsbevordering b.v.

Macdonald, G. (1996) Indicateurs de Qualité et Efficacité de la Promotion de la Santé: la Nécessité de les Marier. Communication, 3ème Conférence Européenne sur l'Efficacité en Promotion de la Santé et en Education pour la Santé, 12–14 September, Turin (unpublished paper).

Miermans, M.C. (1995) Evaluation du Projet 'Agir en Prévention' Brussels: report for the Ministry of Health, unpublished report, APES: 47.

Ovretveit, J. (1994) All together now. *Health Services Journal* December, 24–26.

Ovretveit, J. (1996) Quality in health promotion, *Health Promotion International* 11, 1: 55–62.

Roland, M. and Jamoulle, M. (1995) L'Assurance de Qualité en Médecine Générale, un Concept Ancien. *Patient Care* 23–32.

Taylor, V. (1990) Health education: a theoretical mapping, *Health Education Journal* 49, 1: 12–14.

Tones, K. (1992) Measuring success in health promotion, *Hygie*, 9: 10–14.

Windsor, R.A. *et al.* (1984) *Evaluation of Health Education and Health Promotion Programmes.* Palo Alto: Mayfield Publishing Company, 389.

Wright, C. and Whittington, D. (1992) *Quality Assurance: an Introduction for Health Care Professionals.* London: Churchill Livingstone.

Chapter 9

Quality measures and evaluation of Healthy City policy initiatives

The Liverpool experience

Jane Springett

INTRODUCTION

The Healthy Cities initiative was originally an attempt by WHO/Euro to implement the Health For All (HFA) strategy and health promotion programme through bypassing national governments and implementing HFA at a local level and in a specific setting, in this case, the city (Curtice and McQueen,1990). The resulting Healthy Cities Project has had a major influence on the development of a settings approach towards health policy and health programmes, and has gained root worldwide in a variety of forms. It has spawned a vast range of community based projects and a huge variety of health promotion work from small scale undertakings to the development of healthy public policy at a city wide level (Poland,1996).

This chapter will focus on the latter aspect of the 'Healthy Cities' approach, that of a single healthy city initiative at the local policy level. It will argue that a different approach to evaluation from those currently used in the health sciences is required when developing comprehensive approaches to health promotion through healthy public policy: one grounded in the reality of the policy development process. Having identified the key issues in the development of quality measures of effectiveness, it will demonstrate how the reality of policy-making has an impact on the development of those measures. It will document the experience of grappling with these issues in practice by outlining the way the evaluation of the Liverpool Healthy City Plan evolved using as a framework for analysis the notion of the policy cycle developed by Rist (1994). The difficulties in developing measures of quality and effectiveness will be illustrated demonstrating how pragmatic decisions have to be made when faced with the complex interaction between different activities as well as engaging those responsible for policy development. It will also make visible the real life messiness of a process that at the time of writing is still underway. Finally it will reflect on the relationship between reality and the theory of good evaluation and the lessons that can be learnt from the Liverpool experience.

HEALTH AND HEALTHY CITIES

Local interpretations of what healthy cities/communities means varies. Commonly healthy cities/communities health promoters support a holistic and socio-ecological view of health as opposed to a behavioural approach (Bruce *et al.*, 1995). Health, it is argued, can only be promoted by recognising the inter-relationships between mind, body and spirit, individual and community, global, community and physical systems. The original idea comes from a model developed in the 1980s by Hancock and Perkins which emphasised looking at those inter-relationships in what they called the Mandala of Health (Hancock, 1993). More recently, the model has been developed by Labonte who characterises a healthy city as one which balances health, environment and the economy in a way that is viable and equitable and, most importantly, is sustainable (Labonte,1993). Underlying the approach therefore is a commitment to issues of equity and social justice. Another cornerstone is the involvement of both the community and other non-health sectors in decision-making on health, particularly municipal authorities through their decisions concerning employment, education, housing, water and air pollution and poverty (Blackman, 1995).

Much of the work is effectively invisible, requiring a shift in culture and attitudes. Issues of accountability driven by governmental concerns with controlling public expenditure, and the consequent drive towards managerialism with its emphasis on robust review and control mechanisms (Henkel, 1991), has led to pressure to produce concrete results (Low, 1994). What is expected by a 'Healthy City approach', however, is not clearcut. While the overall vision is a healthier city or community and the Ottawa Charter on Health Promotion (WHO, 1986) is usually the framework for action, the actual manifestation of the approach locally and each project's specific aims and objectives, reflects local concerns, local commitment and local constraints as well as national and cultural differences (Simpson,1994). For some, it is part of broader based pressures for change that uses a vision to raise people from everyday reality to see possibilities. In this it has the characteristics of a social movement albeit with bureaucratic tendencies (Stevenson and Burke, 1991; Baum,1993). For others, it is often seen as health promotion with a community focus (Poland, 1996). At its most developed it can be about co-ordinated planning and healthy public policy (Goumans, 1997; Goumans and Springett, 1997). It is the latter which is the focus of this chapter.

ISSUES IN THE DEVELOPMENT OF QUALITY MEASURES AND EVALUATION OF PUBLIC HEALTH POLICY

The nature of the policy process

Policy development is an iterative and dynamic process involving a range of actors linked together through a network of activities, decisions and motivations

(Klijn, 1992; Considine, 1995). Policy is not a specific decision or intervention (Allison, 1971; Hogwood and Gunn, 1984), policy is produced in, with, and through negotiations between participants. Thus, in practice, there is often no distinction between policy development and implementation, policy is often developed while being implemented (Lipsky, 1980). Changing public policy is notoriously difficult (Siler-Wells, 1987), policy maintenance is more the norm (Pettigrew *et al.*, 1992). If policy change does take place, most of the times it occurs (especially at local level) by incremental steps (Nocon, 1990).

How the actual development of policy manifests itself therefore, depends on local context, and evaluation of its quality and effectiveness will depend on local priorities, constraints and stakeholders. Both are parallel and emergent learning processes for those concerned. Political context and personal preferences, moreover, will affect the direction and utilisation of the evaluation process (Patton, 1982). Much will depend on the theory underlying the policy. This affects what can be evaluated, how it is evaluated and what action will be taken in response (Chen, 1990; Downie *et al.*, 1990). Interpretation of any data and the action chosen will differ in the case where there is an underlying assumption held by policy-makers that ill health is related to lifestyles of individuals (victim-blaming) as opposed to a view that factors outside the control of individuals (such as poverty), are responsible. Much will depend as well on the stories behind the policies, power struggles, personality conflicts and feelings of mutual distrust.

Much also depends on whether a top-down or bottom-up perspective on policy is adopted. Most policy-makers working within current institutional frameworks adopt a top-down perspective, so embedded are Weberian ideas about hierarchical organisation and management (Barrett and Fudge, 1981). This can best be illustrated by a specific example relevant to healthy cities, joint working or intersectoral collaboration. The effectiveness of joint working is as much about the outcomes of joint working as the process by which this outcome has been achieved. One could argue therefore that joint working is effective if it facilitates the desired change (outcome) with the best possible use of working together (process), and that it brings about 'more' change for health – in terms of quality as well as in quantity – than single organisations would have achieved on their own or in other ways. However, effectiveness is a value laden concept and is as much about perceived cost benefits as objective indicators. As with all evaluation, it also depends on who is defining the criteria of effectiveness (Springett *et al.*, 1995). Different perspectives place a different emphasis on process and outcomes depending on whether they take a top-down view or a bottom-up approach to effectiveness.

A planner taking a top-down perspective may assess the process in terms of a good administration structure, perfect co-ordination and measurable goal performance (Sanderson, 1990). This would be seen within the context of the local political and economic situation, and national government policy which can have an impact on the opportunities for effective joint working. Typical in such an assessment is the emphasis on compatible and consistent goals for joint working, reviewing the structures through which it operates and controlling the decision-making process. Issues of participation, for example, would not be considered central to the process and therefore of marginal concern.

For those acting as reticulists (Friend *et al.*, 1974; Hanf and O'Toole, 1992) and taking a bottom-up perspective, effective joint working has all to do with good communication and inter-personal skills, and issues such as trust, mutual respect, openness about self-interest, and the ability to learn from others take priority. Joint working is seen as a process of negotiation between the people involved and an interchange of their beliefs and values. It has as its central concern dialogue and participation. From this perspective, a focus on clear goals and adequate control neglects the underlying processes that influence effective joint working (Sanderson, 1990) since well co-ordinated joint working is not necessarily effective in accomplishing its mission (Butterfoss *et al.*, 1993).

It is from the latter perspect that the joint working experience of the task groups that developed the Liverpool City Health Plan were evaluated by Costongs and Springett (1997a). It was also the approach used by Speller and Furnell (1994) to develop a generic set of indicators for planning, evaluating and creating healthier alliances. In both cases measures of quality and effectiveness are defined in terms of the underlying processes and the processes themselves are seen as valid outcomes. This contrasts with the alternative hierarchical perspective whereby quality and effectiveness are implicitly defined in terms of structure and quantifiable outcomes. The tension between these two perspectives lies at the heart of the evaluation debate and is reflected in the case study below.

The search for indicators

Considerable time and effort has been spent in trying to develop generic indicators for measuring a 'healthy city'. This process has been characterised as a search for the holy grail and is akin to the fruitless search for the ultimate indicator of health (Mootz, 1986). It is possible to draw on the wide range of indicators already available to measure almost any dimension of health-related policy concepts (O'Neill, 1993). However, as the above example illustrates, indicator development cannot be undertaken in isolation from the political and philosophical basis behind the specific health-related policy to be evaluated nor its own unique aims and objectives. Effectiveness analysis has to address the question of whether a policy and its associated programmes have achieved their intended goals and objectives (Schalock, 1995). Indicators will also vary according to who requests the indicators to be selected, who paid for such a selection, who uses it and their specific agendas (O'Neill, 1993). Hence, the process of developing and using indicators to evaluate healthy public policy is more a political problem than a technical one, dependent on world views and power structures, including the ability to impose certain opinions on others (O'Neill, 1993; Baum, 1995). Crucially, the theories concerning health that underpin the policy will drive the process (Chen, 1990). In the Liverpool case study those involved in the development of indicators for measuring change shared as a common theory the socio-ecological model of health and attributed the causes of ill health to the relative poverty and deprivation created by long term unemployment and economic decline. It is perhaps significant that the focus was on the causes of ill health after the salutogenic perspective embodied in the notion: 'the determinants of health'. The search for measurable specific health outcome indicators tends to be driven by a positivist model of research on health which takes as its starting point disease and mortality and the randomised control trial, a reference point to some extent dictated by medical hegemony (Springett and Leavey, 1995). Identifying the effectiveness of health promotion interventions is based on what is measurable, usually quantitatively, what is controllable and what is generalisable. As a result policy analysis is driven often more by a preference for technique (e.g. cost–benefit analysis, survey research, multiple regression, system analysis, etc.), than by the underlying theory upon which the techniques are based (O'Neill and Pederson, 1992). Also rarely do policy-makers develop a set of standards or criteria by which the policy-making process itself is judged.

The positivist paradigm, in which logical-deductive, quantitative measurements and a value-free objectivist science are highly rated is reflected in the current emphasis on evidence-based practice, performance indicators and economic appraisal in the health sector (DOH, 1995). The latter are essentially managerial tools for resource control whereby managers are seen as central actors in the policy process (Considine, 1995). Implicit is the assumption that such systems of performance measurement are sources of policy improvement and that this can be achieved by managers alone without reference to other actors in the process or to external changes (Considine, 1995, p. 248) The dominance of these two ideologies can have a substantial impact on what measurements are chosen and the priorities for developing quality measures for monitoring performance. This has been the case in Liverpool where, although faced with adopting an ecological approach to change, the indicators chosen reflected traditional medical norms and managerial outcomes.

However rigorously designed, evaluations will not influence the policy process just because they are scientific, objective or valid. According to Rist (1994), this linear relation of evaluation to action does not exist. In practice, the real world of policy-making and implementation often throws up conditions which resist positivist methods since policy systems are complex structures for political learning comprising many subcultures and values (Considine, 1995; Weiss, 1988). It is important to consider the values, aspirations and motivations of the people involved, which cannot be quantified (de Leeuw, 1989; Ziglio, 1991). What is required is a flexible, negotiated and process-oriented approach to the evaluation of urban healthy public policy which is more in keeping with the nature of the policy process. This does not mean that outcome measures, qualitative or quantitative, are abandoned, but that all the participants in the process are encouraged to enter into a dialogue, about what is appropriate and possible, thus encouraging reflection on existing perspectives and ideologies. Collaboration, participation and equity are not only central to quality but also to the way quality measures are developed.

The evaluation process

Ideally, what is required is a clear but flexible framework for evaluation that allows for systematic reflection on progress towards achieving aims and objectives, timely and useful information feedback on progress and the opportunity for knowledge development and change (Table 9.1). This iterative

Table 9.1 A framework for the evaluation of local healthy public policy

Step 1	Environmental mapping to provide context and background
Step 2	Establish the purpose of the evaluation
Step 3	Design the evaluation protocol
Step 4	Decide whether or not to use standardised indicators
Step 5	Carry out the data collection
Step 6	Interpret the data obtained
Step 7	Give feedback to all people involved
Step 8	Undertake the actions derived from the evaluation findings

process that, if undertaken systematically, follows a series of steps that highlight a series of decisions that need to be made. The process should also be a cyclical one which follows previous decisions to be revised in the light of new circumstances, that includes the revision of the original aims and objectives and the measures or indicators. Costongs and Springett (1997b) have developed a framework for the evaluation of health related policies using Rist's notion of the policy cycle. Rist (1994) characterises the policy cycle as consisting of three phases, namely: policy formulation, policy implementation and policy accountability (outcome). There is some disagreement amongst policy researchers about whether formulation, implementation and outcome should be isolated as three separate processes, since policy is shaped while being implemented (Hupe, 1990; O'Toole, 1986) and in complex policy situations it is difficult to isolate the relationship between specific policies and specific outcomes. Barrett and Fudge (1981) have talked about a policy-action continuum, without making a distinction between the different phases. Sabatier (1986) however argues that obliterating the distinction between policy formulation and implementation precludes policy evaluation and the analysis of change; as there is never a defined policy which changes into another defined policy. As previously argued much depends on whether a top-down or bottom-up perspective on policy is adopted.

In practice too, most policy evaluation starts well into the policy cycle. This was the case in Liverpool which only relatively recently agreed an evaluation framework. However, implicit in this approach is that in order to improve the quality and effectiveness of health policy, the process of evaluation must become an integral part of the activity of policy development and based on an action research approach (Springett and Leavey, 1995; Gustavsen, 1992; Winter, 1990). Such an approach developed incrementally in Liverpool, but became increasingly accepted as the norm to the extent that it was acknowledged that the set of indicators by which the progress of the city plan would be measured would themselves change over time as priorities changed within the policy cycle.

Participation

There is now therefore a move away in some sectors from a reliance on rigid 'scientific' methodologies, to more interpretative, process-oriented methods with an emphasis on learning from experience which is a feature of the action research approach (for example, Fetterman *et al.*, 1996; Hoggart *et al.*, 1994; Knox and McAlister, 1994; Mathison, 1994; Winje and Hewell, 1992; Barnekov *et al.*, 1990; Means and Smith, 1988; Fuerstein, 1986). This reflects an increasing concern for the variability in evaluation utilisation as well as the failure to develop useful indicators using conventional approaches. Another concern has been the high failure rate of policy implementation in the public services. This failure rate is even higher when intersectoral collaboration is involved (Gray, 1985). Such an approach to evaluation is seen as a prerequisite to ensuring sustainability. It serves both as a management tool to enable people to improve their efficiency and effectiveness and as an educational process in which the participants increase their awareness and understanding of factors which affect their situation. It also ensures the lessons learnt are by those involved in the project locally rather than outsiders. Evaluation itself becomes an agent of change, particularly when it is participatory; research shows that participatory decision-making is the key to sustainable change (Senge, 1990).

The quality of measures developed to monitor and assess effectiveness is therefore directly linked to the process by which they are developed and the degree of participation by key stakeholders in the process. On the grounds of consistency with the principles of intersectoral collaboration and community participation inherent in the 'Healthy City' way of working alone this would seem necessary. But it is also necessary for the effective implementation of any plans or programmes. Unless there is continual feedback between evaluation, planning and activity, improvements in quality are unlikely to take place unless those involved own the information and the process (Patton, 1982). This is particularly important where a complex multilevel approach to change focuses on the long term (Goodman *et al.*, 1996). Only by taking people through the decision-making process on what questions to ask and how they can be effectively answered are unrealistic demands concerning short term outcome measurement likely to be moderated. Knowledge development is a key feature of the process, as is the importance of opening up channels of communication within the policy process (Sarri and Sarri, 1992; Cousins and Earl, 1992; Winje and Hewell, 1992). Policy-makers often do not have direct first-hand knowledge of the problems they are called upon to solve. On the other hand, the implementors who know these problems, do not have enough power to adjust and improve this policy. Similarly, the beneficiaries of the policy may hold key information and be a resource in finding solutions as well a vital element in assessing policy effectiveness (De Koning and Martin, 1996).

Participatory approaches also actively encourage collaboration. But it also means that what is evaluated and how and with what measures will be a reflection of who is actually involved in the process. By implication, if you go through that same process with a different group of people there is a probability that a different outcome will be achieved, a different set of policy choices made and a different set of measures of change (Gustavsen, 1992; Hazen, 1994). On the other hand, account can be made of the conditions favouring and impeding the policy process within the city (Ziglio, 1991) such as what structures and processes make it possible to achieve changes in the complex urban environment (Tsouros and Draper, 1993).

In participatory evaluation there is dialogue and feedback at every stage. There is constant feedback into the policy process, so reality is a moving target and changing constantly. Participants will be altered by the process as it proceeds too, as they learn from reflection on their experiences in policy development. Stakeholders in being part of the process find their assumptions, their practices and perceptions being challenged (Radaelli, 1995). It requires them to devote time and commitment to actually reflect and since many policy-makers and decision-makers are task oriented this can initially be seen as alien or even unnecessary. On the other hand involvement creates a strong ownership of the knowledge and information that emerges as part of the process and stakeholders are more likely to put into practice what that information reveals. This is the essence of capacity building. Finally, there are consequences for the way things are measured. Decisions concerning evaluation design and methodology become eclectic leading to the use of a combination of quantitative and qualitative techniques.

Belief in the information gained in assessing effectiveness is increased when people 'own' the results and understand them, which is enhanced by their involvement in the process of evaluation (Patton, 1982). Public participation is therefore as important as involving policy-makers. Those who are affected by a policy initiative are the people who know the problem intimately and how to act upon them. However, in practice, it has proved as difficult to involve city inhabitants in evaluation as it has in political decision-making. Local people become frustrated with the lack of action on matters that concern them and can be unwilling to participate (Quellet *et al.*, 1994). People will get involved only when they see a glimmer of a solution or when they feel empowered. This is probably the greatest challenge to the healthy city movement in terms of policy development. Conventional bureaucratic structures do not lend themselves well to democratic involvement as the Liverpool case study will show.

THE LIVERPOOL EXPERIENCE

The final part of this chapter will outline how Liverpool tackled the evaluation of its City Health Plan. The process has been a learning experience for all concerned and is a continuing one as each stage of reflection is reached. At the time of writing, the policy context of the local health strategy is changing rapidly following a change in national government, stimulating a re-examination of aims and objectives, local priorities and action. Certain key stakeholders have been influential in influencing the way evaluation has evolved, while the limited resources available for evaluation has dictated a patchwork quilt or jigsaw approach to data collection and the relative involvement of internal and external evaluators. Pragmatism and changing perspectives as both the evaluation and the policy process have evolved have also influenced the types of decisions made. In essence it has been a case study of continuous quality improvement applied to healthy public policy. It also has been a slow development process. After providing some key background information, the evaluation process will be discussed using Rist's policy cycle as an organising framework.

The socio-economic, political and organisational context

Liverpool is a deprived city in the United Kingdom with approximately 477,000 inhabitants that has suffered the consequences of an economic recession, due to the decline of its port and associated industries. A Quality of Life Survey shows poverty undertaken in 1991 at twice the national average with an unemployment rate of 21.6 per cent. However there is wide variation within the city from 8.5 per cent to 36.7 per cent. This level of deprivation has meant it was given Objective 1 status by the EU for the purposes of regional economic development. It also is the recipient of a number of substantial redevelopment grants and funds from national government. The allocation of these grants is in some cases, directly linked to the requirement of involving the public and multiagency partnerships. Alongside such development community health forums have been created to provide a voice for those who feel unable to influence decision-makers. There are also a large number of voluntary agencies whose remit covers health related concerns. However, not withstanding this the key central players in the development of the city health strategy audits evaluations have been the local authority and the health authority, both of whom dominate the city in terms of employment, resources and decision-making on public policy. There is a long history of state involvement in economic development and the provision of services in the city. The long-standing structural and organisational arrangements influence policy and decision-making and this can frustrate attempts at more open systems approaches to development (Dugdill *et al.*, 1997),

Liverpool has been involved in the WHO Healthy City project since its inception in 1987. In the first five years of the project, in common with many other cities, it failed to move beyond small scale model project development to healthy public policy, although the groundwork was laid for more effective coalition working in the second phase (Goumans and Springett, 1997). Changes of personnel and a commitment from the local health authorities to work together more closely heralded a new phase of development in 1993, the central plank of which was the development of a City Health plan of strategy. The latter was a key requirement of the membership of the second phase of the WHO/Euro project.

A Joint Public Health Team was established in 1993 to lead the development of the plan accountable to the Joint Consultative Committee. It was separate from existing traditional joint care planning arrangements involving mainly social and health service providers. In addition there is also a Healthy City unit to provide administration and support for joint public health working between the agencies in the city and the community. In order to formulate and write the strategies for the plan, four task groups were specifically set up to address key areas of the UK government *Health of the Nation* document (1992) (heart disease, cancer, sexual health and accidents) as well as one task group on 'housing for health'. Following the production of the plan the task groups were disbanded. Implementation was now seen as the remit of existing organisations and their departmental managers. The Joint Public Health team would retain an overview of ongoing developments and monitoring and evaluation. The Healthy City Unit's role is to support the team in that process and facilitate implementation.

The draft City Health Plan was launched in January 1995; this was followed by a five month consultation process and revision of the plan leading to its publication in 1996. The Plan is the Health Authority's five year strategy and a corporate priority within the City Council. In its broadest terms the plan aims to influence, co-ordinate and integrate purchasing, service and business planning in the city. It makes strong links with other city wide initiatives that focus on economic and social regeneration action. The focus of implementation, however, is through local area partnerships in the most disadvantaged areas of the city. It explicitly tackles the underlying causes of ill health, namely the environment, the economy including poverty and unemployment, housing, education, crime and transport (Taylor, 1997). Specific action is aimed at smoking, nutrition and physical activity and particular population groups:

children and young people, black and other ethnic minorities and older people. It also sought targets in the Health of the Nation areas of heart disease, cancer, mental health, sexual health and accidents. Its explicit mission is: 'That in five years time there will be an improvement in the quality of life and health of everyone, particularly those people in Liverpool experiencing poverty and disadvantage.' (Liverpool Healthy City 2000, 1996.)

The nature of the evaluation process in Liverpool

In the first phase of the policy cycle, evaluation is needed to understand and to define clearly the health related issue. Such formative evaluation also should allow reflection on possible policy options as well as the constraints that policy-makers are faced with. Collecting such baseline information is a lengthy process so in practice the process of information collection usually takes place in tandem with policy formulation or even afterwards. Plans are static but policies are constantly evolving so when the city health plan was finally launched in 1996 it was already in the stages of implementation. Minutes of the JPHT meetings reveal a constant willingness to reflect and modify approaches as feedback was received, revealing a tangential process of development and evaluation taking place. For as Rist (1994, p. 549) noted: 'the window for policy formulation is frequently very small and open only a short time. The information that can be passed through has to be ready and in a form that enhances quick understanding'.

In Liverpool the development of the City Health plan drove the process in the first cycle of this place. In the second cycle of this phase, the implementation of the plan and changes in the policy context led to a re-examination of priorities in the light of new policy options.

Evaluation in phase 1 largely involved understanding and defining the key health issues rather than a systematic review of the policy options. Information and data collection was based on intuitive understanding and experience and collective knowledge as well as existing research, providing a multilevel collection of qualitative and quantitative data, some systematically collected, others related to the stories people held in their heads (Taylor, 1997). The Health of the Nation provided the policy window but policy-makers built on the experience developed in the first five years of the project. This understanding then was measured qualitatively against community experience during the consultation process, as well as through the bringing together of existing mapped data. Existing policies and programmes were also mapped at the time highlighting when co-ordination between these policies was needed. The aims and objectives were modified as a result of this process. This geographical approach to the need assessment stage was a significant influence on the nature of the final strategy. The information gained was also fed back into the decision-making processes of the City Council and the Health Authority, leading to an active focus on the most disadvantaged areas of the city. It also fed into the grand applying process that has become a feature of resource generation within the city. Regeneration overall became a focus of health policy.

It was quite clear by the end of this process that there would be two dimensions to the strategy. First, a geographical approach to policy implementation would be taken, focusing on key areas within the city which consistently demonstrated low scores on a range of key health related indexes taken from the consensus and would influence action areas within different sectors of policy. Second, there would be an attempt to influence decision-makers in the city in the key sectors identified by the task group process and the consultation process.

The City Health plan was essentially a joint plan between the Health and Local Authorities. The process itself led to the development of a good relationship between these two authorities at a strategic level but also placed an emphasis on a top-down and managerial approach to policy. What is clear is that the parties concerned already shared a similar theory of health and its promotion, firmly grounded in a socio-ecological model of change, building strongly on existing theories of the relationship between health and unemployment. It was this model, together with existing priorities, which drove the plan development. The participants did not share the national government's disease and victim blaming lifestyle model of health, but were forced by circumstance to follow that model in development. It was clear that although an attempt was made to fit into the disease model, the final plan came back to the underlying causes of ill health, as in their planning, the task groups overlapped in their solutions to the problems they identified. This view was reinforced by the outcomes of the consultation process whereby further information gained led to a revamping of the plan, raising environment up the agenda. The environment had not been priority with the main authorities, however it was one for the community (Taylor, 1997).

The final plan therefore was a product of the information gained during its formulation but also of the dominance of certain stakeholders in the decision-making process. Participation in decision-making in plan development focused largely around the task groups and through the consultation process. Both processes were evaluated externally using resources from the two local Universities (Costongs and Springett, 1997a; Strobl and Bruce, 1997). The membership of the task groups comprised purchasers of services and consumers. A total of 160 people worked on the production of the City Health Plan. The organisations represented were: the city council (social services, environmental health, education), health authority, community health councils, age concern, universities, health promotion agency, trades council and several voluntary groups. This approach contrasts with that adopted in Sheffield which started with needs assessment at the grass roots (Healthy Sheffield Development Unit, 1993). Part of the explanation for this lies in the timeline set to produce the plan but also in the bureaucratic tradition within Liverpool. Only after a draft plan had been produced where categories had already been defined for action was the plan put out for consultation.

Community participation was achieved through the five month consultation process, itself generating new information and leading to changes in policy focus. Given the complexity of the city plan with its focus on such a wide range of sectors consultation represented a challenge in operational terms. The ideal was to combine successfully highly complex areas of higher level strategic planning with wider participation to guide those activities. To do this the language and concerns of day to day life have to be integrated with the bigger picture and all need to learn from one another. What made the consultation process unique at the time, was the fact it was the most resourced to date and that it used largely new and innovative sets of methods. Moreover, there was a genuine willingness of key stakeholders to enter into dialogue with the community (Strobl and Bruce, 1997).

The consultation process began with a public launch in January 1995 followed by encouragement to comment through newspaper inserts, public posters, radio broadcasts, and mailing of an abridged version of the plan to every household in Liverpool. The main method, however, was the use of fifty-three trained facilitators from the statutory and voluntary sectors who were available to hold group meetings, supported by a video. The full evaluation of the process is presented elsewhere (Strobl and Bruce, 1997) and focuses only on the consultation process of the draft plan. No evaluation was undertaken as to whether the final plan met the concerns of the community who participated.

This failure to look at evaluation systematically, to identify what should be evaluated and how it could be fed into the process was a key feature of this early phase. The external evaluation which did take place was the product of university driven concerns and related to the availability of appropriate resources. The evaluation work focused on process indicators and both were qualitative studies. Information concerning the joint working was immediately fed back into the process and actively led to a review of joint care planning but no specific action for eighteen months. The consultation review was only available one year after it took place. It is difficult to identify specific process changes although reference is made then to the reports in meetings. The lack of involvement of the key stakeholders in defining the questions for evaluation may account for the lack of ownership of the results.

Policy implementation

The focus in the second phase of the policy-cycle is on the 'day to day realities of bringing a new policy into existence' (Rist, 1994). Intersectoral polices are notorious for failing to be implemented (Gray, 1985). Evaluation of key aspects of this process can act as an early warning and actively encourage the process of change. Questions of interest here include: Is the policy being implemented as planned? (Pirie, 1990). Have new formal or informal interorganisational networks developed? (Milio, 1986). Is there enough institutional capacity and expertise to respond effectively to the new policy, if this policy is accepted by the implementing officials? What aspects of the policy are not operational? Since target populations and conditions related to health within a city are changing continuously, an ongoing and process-orientated evaluation helps implementors to match and adjust their activities to the present circumstances. Some of these questions are only just beginning to be addressed in Liverpool. The failure to engage in systematic evaluation was only actively addressed by the key strategic stakeholders in the year following the launch of the plan and is still a feature of ongoing debate. The JPHT became for a time very task driven and its agenda crowded with operational items and presentations on action being taken. Lack of clarity concerning their strategic role together with a desire to let go of the plan during its implementation phase contributed to this hiatus. The issue of evaluation was raised with the team a number of times, both as a presentation and a paper presented at two different meetings (JPHT, 1996). In that paper it was suggested that the evaluation process should be used to extend both participation in the decision-making process and implementation to middle managers who had not been party to the development of the plan and yet were expected to deliver its contents.

To move the debate forward a series of workshops took place. In the first, aims and objectives of the plan were revisited and priorities identified. In the second, the focus was on indicators (see below). In the third the focus was on one of the key aims of the health for all movement, community participation. Eventually a framework emerged that now drives the evaluation and monitoring process. A significant achievement has been the placing of health issues on the agendas of the evaluation of the partnership areas (Tables 9.2 and 9.3). The Healthy City Unit has been a key player in making this happen.

As in the first phase, pragmatic use of external resources has added pieces to the jigsaw including an audit of service plan within the city council to identify whether they are implementing the city health plan. The information gained is being used at a workshop for key managers within the city council. A studentship was used to collect qualitative information on the reach of the ideas in the strategy amongst middle managers and those lead managers who are not currently part of the core team. The development of a system of regular reporting of achievements and failures has been instituted. Again the concerns have been driven by the two key stakeholders who dominate the decision-making process. Involvement of other agencies has been limited, as has community participation. At the time of writing the realisation of the need for a more systematic approach to evaluation has however finally been accepted and a plan is evolving to replace *ad hoc* evaluation with an evaluation process that has as its context a clear view of aims and objectives.

Policy outcome

Another reason that the issue of a broad and systematic approach to evaluation was slow to be addressed was the overriding concern of key stakeholders

Table 9.2 *Priority 1: community safety* (operational objective: to highlight the health aspects of and develop constructive links with other elements of the overall regeneration strategy for the Speke Garston area)

Objective	Those involved	Lead	Target and timescale
To raise awareness of the importance of community safety as a key factor in improving the emotional and physical health of local people by including this perspective in health promotion activities and campaigns	Health Co-ordination Group, Health Forum, Community Safety Co-ordinator, Health Promotion	Neighbourhood Health Development Project	December 1998
To ensure that improved emotional and physical health is recognised as an important outcome of enhanced community safety within the Partnership's Community Safety Strategy	Health Forum, Health Co-ordination Group, Community Safety Working Group	Speke Partnership, Garston	July 1997
To support the implementation of the action points in the Partnership's Community Safety Strategy, particularly those which have a significant impact on health, including measures to reduce traffic accidents, helping victims of crime and improved street lighting	Health Forum, Health Co-ordination Group, Merseyside Police, Victim Support	Speke Partnership, Garston	Timescale dependent on Community Safety Strategy
To draw particular attention to the safety of young children in preventing accidents and accidents in the home	Health Forum, Health visitors, City Council planning and transportation	—	Timescale dependent on Community Safety Strategy
To improve the safety of play areas	Health Forum, City Council youth services	City Council Education Department	December 1998

Table 9.3 Priority 2: addressing poverty and unemployment as major underlying causes of ill health (operational objective: to highlight the health aspects of, and develop constructive linkages with other elements of the overall regeneration strategy for the Speke Garston area)

Objective	Those involved	Lead	Target and timescale
To provide a range of anti-poverty services and activities in the Partnership area including: welfare rights information, advice and advocacy, Credit Union services including the development of bill-paying facilities	Citizens Advice Bureau, Speke Community Credit Union, Community Groups	Speke Partnership, Garston	Ongoing
To investigate ways in which low-cost furniture and household equipment can be provided in the area to add to the service provided by CREATE	CREATE, Furniture Resource Centre Business Link, Speke Garston Partnership	Speke Partnership, Garston	Feasibility study completed by November 1997
To facilitate the provision of low-cost shopping relevant to people's needs at key points in the area, particularly Garston Village and Speke District Centre	Private Sector, Speke Garston Partnership, Inner City Enterprises, Liverpool City Council	Speke Partnership, Garston	According to timescales of Garston Regeneration Strategy and Speke District Centre Implementation Plan
To implement strategies which will achieve inward investment and employment and enable local people to access employment and training	Private Sector, Speke Garston Partnership, Speke Garston Development Company, Merseyside TEC, agencies involved in training and development	Speke Partnership, Garston	According to timescales of Partnership Delivery Plan

to measure policy outcome. 'How will we know we have made a difference?' was the key question that emerged from early workshops for the JPHT. As a result, considerable time, energy and resources were spent on finding and developing key quantifiable indicators. A review of health indicators was commissioned, a workshop was held involving local experts and city council resources were devoted to reviewing the information currently collected in the areas covered by the plan. In common with other attempts to find good quality quantifiable and resource efficient indicators the results were disappointing. The framework for the development of that search is shown in Figures 9.1 and 9.2 where the problem of linking cause to outcome is demonstrated (Willis, 1996). The outcome of that process is reported in the 1996 Public Health Annual Report (Liverpool Health Authority, 1997) (Table 9.4). What that report reveals is how limited current indicators are when examining health rather than disease outcomes (Lucy, 1996). It also makes suggestions as to future data collection, including a health and well-being survey, which is being piloted in one of the partnership areas (Christakopoulou and Dawson, 1997).

The outcome of the process of developing indicators may have been disappointing in terms of its original objectives but what has been achieved is the challenging of assumptions concerning what should make good indicators leading to: (1) a decision to balance quantifiable indicators with qualitative ones; (2) a recognition of the difficulty in developing indicators that truly reflect the web of causality which the city health plan tried to address; (3) an acknowledgement of those factors over which there is no control and may actually reduce the chances of achieving the aims and objectives of the plan; (4) a search for new approaches to notions of health gain and health impact; (5) an increasing acceptance that the measurement of progress cannot rely on indicators that bear little resemblance to the aims and objectives of the plan; (6) an acknowledgement of the need to look at process as well as outcome; (7) an acceptance of the key role of the JPHT in making connections and evaluating and monitoring the implementation process. Interestingly, similar conclusions are represented in research literature; the JPHT, however, needed to go through the learning process itself and was only tangentially conscious of what research was telling them.

COMMENTARY

This chapter has demonstrated how the evaluation process has contributed to the development of quality measures related to health policy in Liverpool. Policy-makers find it difficult to face up to criticism and the nature of the policy process is such that it is a complex learning exercise involving many actors (Minogue, 1983; Radaelli, 1995; Klijn, 1994; Sabatier, 1987). This has been illustrated by concentrating on the learning process the JPHT in

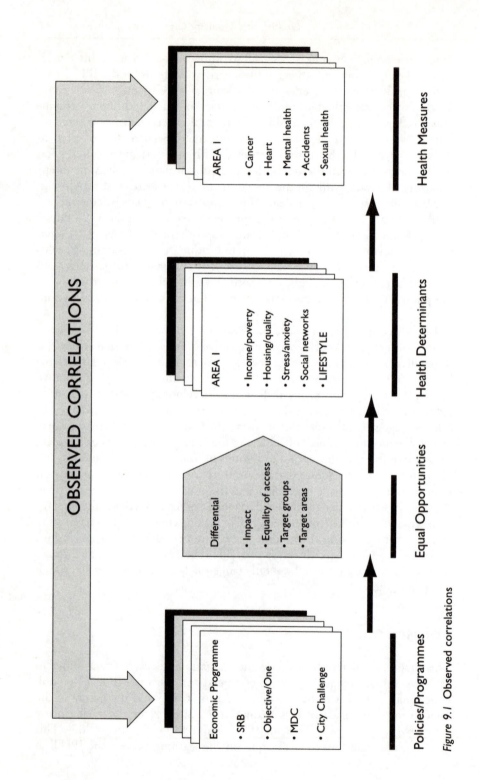

Figure 9.1 Observed correlations

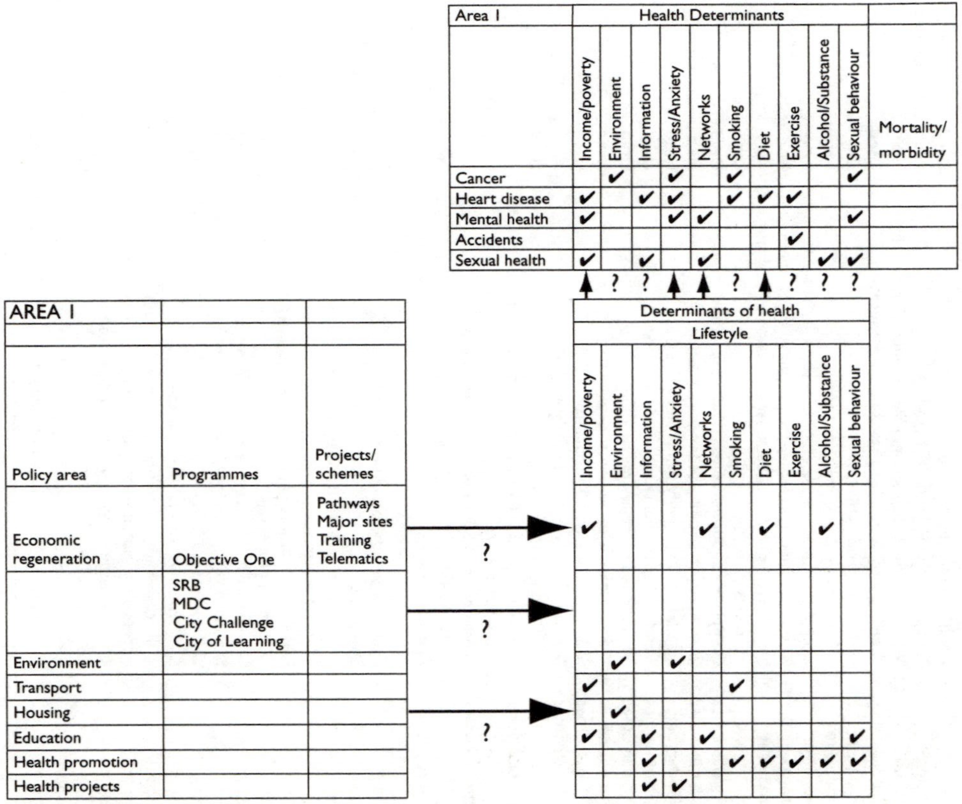

Area I

	Income/poverty	Environment	Information	Stress/Anxiety	Networks	Smoking	Diet	Exercise	Alcohol/Substance	Sexual behaviour	Mortality/morbidity
Health Determinants											
Cancer	✓	✓		✓		✓	✓			✓	
Heart disease	✓		✓	✓		✓	✓	✓			
Mental health				✓	✓					✓	
Accidents									✓		
Sexual health	✓		✓	✓	✓				✓	✓	

Determinants of health — Lifestyle

	Income/poverty	Environment	Information	Stress/Anxiety	Networks	Smoking	Diet	Exercise	Alcohol/Substance	Sexual behaviour
	✓				✓		✓		✓	✓
						✓				✓
	✓	✓	✓	✓						
	✓	✓	✓		✓				✓	✓
			✓	✓						✓

AREA I

Policy area	Programmes	Projects/schemes
Economic regeneration	Objective One SRB MDC City Challenge City of Learning	Pathways Major sites Training Telematics
Environment		
Transport		
Housing		
Education		
Health promotion		
Health projects		

Figure 9.2 Ruptures in the ideal matrix

Table 9.4 Public Health Annual Report 1996

City Health Plan Chapter	Indicator name	Status
Accidents	Pedestrian accidents (0–14) per length of road	Rejected
Accidents	Number of cyclist accidents per length of road	Rejected
Accidents	Car occupants aged 15–24 per length of road	Rejected
Accidents	Hospital admission for accidents	Rejected
Accidents	Deaths from accidents	Rejected
Crime	Burglary against dwelling per 100 residential properties	Used
Crime	Violent crime per 100 night time population	Used
Crime	Arson or damage per 100 properties	Used
Crime	Juvenile disorder per 100 average day time population	Used
Economy	% of economically active people unemployed and claiming benefit	Used
Economy	% of unemployed aged 18–24	Used
Economy	% of unemployed, unemployed for more than a year	Used
Education	% of primary school pupils reaching level 4 in the SATS for English, Maths and Science	Used
Education	% pupils attaining 5+ GCSEs grade A–E	Published elsewhere
Education	% population 17–24 receiving higher education awards	Used
Education	% of 0–5 yr-olds receiving state nursery education	Used
Environment	Nitrogen dioxide pollution	City wide
Environment	% land classified as derelict or vacant	Rejected
Environment	Complaints about refuse collection per 1,000 population	Rejected
Environment	% land classified as green space for public enjoyment	Rejected
Environment	No. of streets graded substandard cleanliness/total length of streets	Used
Health outcomes	Complaints about noise per 1,000 population	Used
Health outcomes	Cancer registration rates for breast cancer	Data awaited
Health outcomes	Standardised mortality ratios all causes 0–74	Used
Health outcomes	Standardised mortality ratios – heart disease	Used
Health outcomes	Standardised mortality ratios – lung cancer	Used
Health outcomes	% 5 year olds with no dental decay	Used
Health outcomes	% 2 year olds with full vaccination	Used
Health outcomes	% babies born with a birth weight of less than 2,500 grammes	Used
Health outcomes	% women aged 25–64 who have had a cervical smear test in the last 5 years	Used
Health outcomes	% women aged 50–64 who have had a breast screening test	Data awaited
Health services	Age standardised emergency admission rates per 100,000 population	Used
Housing	Domestic energy rating (average for area)	Data awaited
Housing	Dampness	Data awaited
Housing	% long-term vacants, demolished or disposed of per 1,000 dwellings	Rejected
Housing	Pest complaints (rats, mice, cockroaches) per 1,000 residential properties	Used
Poverty	% households in receipt of housing benefits	Used
Poverty	% households in receipt of council tax benefits	Used
Poverty	% children aged 5–16 receiving free school meals	Used
Transport	% of crossings with tactile pavements	Data unavailable
Transport	% of roads with bus routes (by length of road)	Rejected
Transport	Accessibility measures for disabled by public transport	Rejected
Transport	% of unclassified roads which have been calmed (by length of road)	Rejected
Transport	% children aged 0–16 within $\frac{1}{4}$ mile of a safe playground	Used
Transport	% of residents within 250m of a bus stop	Used

Liverpool has undergone in developing its own framework for evaluation. Persuading them as to the importance of systematically addressing key concerns and how they should be measured was difficult. One of the key features of that experience is how people changed in terms of perceptions and priorities and how evaluation only gradually rose up the policy agenda. This was essentially a task of capacity building, a key prerequiste for effective decision-making and policy implementation (Goodman *et al.*, 1996). The evaluation process fell short of the systematic ideal and was largely dependent on internal resources although one member of the JPHT was an experienced evaluator and along with the Healthy City Unit attempted to push it up the policy agenda. Their success in doing that was dependent on the learning process outlined. As Fuerstein (1986) has demonstrated internal evaluation alone has both strengths and weaknesses. One of the key features of its strengths is that it encourages learning to take place, one of its weaknesses is that key evaluation questions get overridden by operational concerns. To get the balance right requires the commitment of adequate resources to evaluation. Persuading policy-makers of the importance of this is as difficult as persuading those working on small scale health promotion projects. What is required is a demystification of evaluation as a research task and its acceptance as integral part of change. The challenge is to create learning communities and organisations. Only then will knowledge development occur and good quality measures of effectiveness of health promotion be developed. Evaluation is a process, not a task. Given the complexity of bringing about healthy public policy, it can be nothing less.

REFERENCES

Allison, G. (1971) *Essence of Decision: Explaining the Cuban Missile Crisis.* Boston: Little, Brown and Company.

Barnekov, T., Hart, D. and Benfer, W. (1990) *US Experience in Evaluating Urban Regeneration.* London: HMSO.

Barrett, S. and Fudge, C. (eds) (1981) Examining the policy–action relationship. *Policy and Action*, 65–82.

Baum, F. (1993). Healthy cities and change: social movement or bureaucratic tool? *Health Promotion International* 8(1), 31–40.

Baum, F. (1995) Research and policy to promote health: what's the relationship? In Bruce, N., Springett, J. Hodgekiss, J. and Scott Samuel, A. (eds) *Research and Change in Urban Community Health.* Aldershot: Avebury, 11–31.

Blackman, T. (1995) *Urban Policy in Practice.* London: Routledge.

Bruce, N., Springett, J., Scott- Samuel, A. and Hodgekiss, J. (1995) *Research and Change in Urban Community Health:* Aldershot: Avebury.

Butterfoss, F.D., Goodman, R.M. and Wandersman, A. (1993) Community coalitions for prevention and health promotion. *Health Education Research: Theory and Practice*, 8(3), 315–330.

Chen, H.T. (1990) *Theory-driven Evaluations.* Newbury Park: Sage Publications.

Christakopulou, S. and Dawson, J. (1997) *An instrument for the evaluation of local community well being in European cities.* Unpublished paper. Liverpool John Moores University.

Considine, M. (1995) *Public Policy: a Critical Approach*. London: Macmillan.

Costongs, C. and Springett, J. (1997a) Joint working and the production of a city health plan: the Liverpool experience. *Health Promotion International* 12(1), 9–19.

Costongs, C. and Springett, J. (1997b) Towards a framework for the evaluation of health-related policies in cities. *Evaluation* 3(3), 345–365.

Cousins, J. B. and Earl, L.M. (1992) The case for participatory evaluation. *Educational Evaluation and Policy Analysis* 14(4), 397–418.

Curtice, L. and McQueen, D.V. (1990) *The WHO Healthy City Project: an Analysis of Progress*, Working Paper no. 2, Research Unit in Health and Behavioural Change, University of Edinburgh.

De Koning, K. and Martin, M. (1996) *Participatory Research in Health*. London: Zed Books.

De Leeuw, E. (1989) *Health Policy: an Exploratory Inquiry into the Development of Policy for the New Public Health in the Netherlands*. Maastricht. Savannah.

De Leeuw, E., O'Neill, M., Goumans, M. and de Bruijn, F. (eds) (1992) *Healthy Cities Research Agenda. Proceedings of an Expert Panel*. RHC Monograph Series no. 2. Maastricht University Press.

Dept of Health (1992) *The Health of the Nation*. London: HMSO.

Dept of Health (1995) *Policy Appraisal and Health*. A guide from the Department of Health. London: HMSO.

Downie, R.S., Fyfe, C. and Tannahill, A.(1990) *Health Promotion, Models and Values*. Oxford: Oxford University Press.

Dugdill, L. and Fennessey, M. (1997) *Urban Primary Care Development: Baring Foundation/ King's Fund Development Initiative: Liverpool. An Interim Report in the Evaluation*. Public Health Research and Resource Centre, Salford University.

Fetterman, D.M., Kaftarian, S.J. and Wandersman, A. (eds) (1996) *Empowerment, Evaluation Knowledge and Tools for Self-assessment and Accountability*. Thousand Oaks, California: Sage.

Friend, J.K., Power, J. and Yewlett,C. (1974) *Public Planning: the Intercorporate Dimension*. London: Tavistock.

Fuerstein, M.T. (1986) *Partners in Evaluation*. London: Macmillan.

Goodman, R.M. *et al.* (1996) An ecological assessment of community based interventions for prevention and health promotion: approaches to measuring community coalitions. *American Journal of Community Psychology* 24(1), 33–61.

Goumans, M. (1997) Innovations in a fuzzy domain: healthy cities and health policy development in the Netherlands and the United Kingdom. PhD thesis, University of Maastricht.

Goumans, M. and Springett, J. (1997) From projects to policy: 'Healthy Cities' as a mechanism for policy change for health? *Health Promotion International* 12(4), 311–322.

Gray, B. (1985) Conditions facilitating interorganizational collaboration. *Human Relations*, 38 (10): 911–936.

Gustavsen, B. (1992) *Dialogue and Development*. Assen: Van Gorcum.

Hancock, T. (1993) Health, human development and the community ecosystem: three ecological models. *Health Promotion International* 8(1) 41–47.

Hanf, I.C. and O'Toole, L. (1992) Revisiting old friends: networks, implementation, structures, and the management of organisational relations. *European Journal of Political Research* 2 163–180.

Hazen, M.A. (1994) A radical humanist perspective of interorganisational relationships. *Human Relations* 47(4), 393–415.

Healthy Sheffield Development Unit (1993) *Framework for Action Healthy Sheffield*. Sheffield: Directorate of Environmental Services and Standards.

Henkel, M. (1991) The new evaluative state. *Public Administration* 69 (1), 121–136.

Hoggart, R., Jeffries, S. and Harrison, L. (1994) Reflexivity and uncertainty in the research process. *Policy and Politics* 22(1): 59–70.

Hogwood, B. and Gunn, L. (1984) *Policy Analysis for the Real World*. Oxford: Oxford University Press.

Hupe, P. (1990) Implementing a meta-policy: the case of decentralization in the Netherlands. *Policy and Politics* 18(3), 181–191.

JPHT (1996). Minutes of the Meeting of the Joint Public Health Team, June 6 1996. Unpublished.

Klijn, E. (1992) *Policy Communities, Subsystems and Networks: An Examination and Reformulation of Some Concepts for Analysing Complex Policy Processes*. Research programme: Policy and Governance in Complex Networks Working paper no. 4 Rotterdam/ Leiden: Erasmus University Rotterdam/ Rijksunversiteit Leiden.

Knox, C. and McAlister, D. (1994) Policy evaluation: incorporating user views. *Public Administration* 73, 413–415.

Labonte, R. (1993) Holosphere of healthy and sustainable communities. *Australian Journal of Public Health* 17(1), 119–128.

Lipsky, M. (1980) Streetlevel Bureaucracy: Dilemmas of the Individual in Public Services. New York: Russel Sage Foundation.

Liverpool Healthy City 2000 (1996) *Liverpool City Health Plan*. Liverpool.

Liverpool Health Authority (1997) *Annual Public Health Report 1996*. Liverpool.

Low, C. (1994) Healthy cities: developing models and facing dilemmas: the Queensland Experience, in Chu, C. and Simpson, R. (eds) *Ecological Public Health: from Vision to Practice*. Toronto: Centre for Health Promotion: University of Toronto.

Lucy, J. (1996) *Health Indicators: A Literature Review*. Liverpool: Public Health Observatory, University of Liverpool.

Mathison, S. (1994) Rethinking the evaluator role: partnerships between organisations and evaluators. *Evaluation and Planning* 17(3), 299–304.

Means, R. and Smith, R. (1988) Implementing a pluralistic approach to evaluation in health education. *Policy and Politics*. 16(1), 17–28.

Milio, N. (1986) *Promoting Health through Public Policy*. Ottawa: Canadian Public Health Association.

Minogue, M. (1983) Theory and practice in public policy and administration. *Policy and Politics*. 11, 63–85.

Mootz, M. (1986) Health indicators. *Social Science and Medicine* 22, 255–276.

Nocon, A. (1990) Making a reality of joint planning. *Local Government Studies*, March/April, 55–67.

O'Neill, M. (1993) Building bridges between knowledge and action: the Canadian process of healthy communities indicators. In Davies, J.K. and Kelly, M.P. (eds) *Healthy Cities: Research and Practice*. London: Routledge.

O'Neill, M. and Pederson, A.P. (1992) Building a methods bridge between public policy analysis and healthy public policy. *Canadian Journal of Public Health* Supplement 1, 83, S25–S30.

O'Toole, L.J. (1986) Policy recommendations for multi-actor implementation: an assessment of the field. *Journal of Public Policy*, 6(2), 181–210.

Patton, M.Q. (1982) *Practical Evaluation*. London: Sage.

Pettigrew, A., Ferilie, A. and McKee, L. (1992) *Shaping Strategic Change*. London: Sage.

Pirie, P.L. (1990) Evaluation. In: Bracht, N. (ed.) *Health Promotion at the Community Level*. Newbury Park, Cal.: Sage.

Poland, B. (1996) Knowledge development and evaluation in, of, and for healthy community initiatives. Part 1: guiding principles. *Health Promotion International* 11(3), 237–247.

Quellet, F., Durand, D. and Forget, G. (1994) Preliminary results of an evaluation of three healthy cities initiatives in the Montreal area. *Health Promotion International*. 9(3), 153–159.

Radaelli, C. (1995) The role of knowledge in the policy process. *Journal of European Public Policy* 2, 2, 159–183.

Rist, R. (1994) Influencing the policy process with qualitative research. In Denzin, N. and Lincoln, Y. (eds) *Handbook of Qualitative Research*. London: Sage.

Rootman, I., Goodstadt, M., Potvin, I. and Springett, J. (1997) *A Framework for Health Promotion Evaluation*. A background paper for the WHO/Euro Working Group on Evaluation of Health Promotion Approaches. Copenhagen: WHO/EURO.

Sabatier, P. (1986) Knowledge, policy-oriented learning, and policy change: an advocacy coalition framework. *Knowledge: Creation, Diffusion, Utilization* 8(4), 649–692.

Sanderson, I. (1990) *Effective Inter Sectoral Collaboration: the Theoretical Issues*. Leeds: Health Education Unit, Leeds Metropolitan University.

Sarri, R.C. and Sarri, C.M. (1992) Organisational and community change through participatory action research. *Administration in Social Work* 16(3/4), 99–122.

Schalock, R.L. (1995) *Outcome based evaluation*. New York: Plenum Press.

Senge, P. (1990) *The Fifth Discipline: the Art and the Practice of Organisational Learning*. New York: Doubleday.

Siler-Wells, G. (1987) An implementation model for health system reform. *Social Science and Medicine* 24(10), 821–832.

Simpson, R. (1994) Integration of environmental health into planning for urban development: the Asia Pacific perspective. In Chu, C. and Simpson, R. (eds) *Ecological Public Health: from Vision to Practice*. Toronto: Centre for Health Promotion and ParticipACTION, 260–268.

Speller, V. and Furnell, R. (1994) *HEA Multisectoral Collaboration for Health Evaluative Project Dissemination Pack*. Southampton: Wessex Public Medicine Institute.

Springett, J. and Leavey, C. (1995) Participatory action research: the development of a paradigm: dilemmas and prospects. In Bruce, N., Springett, J. Hodgkiss, J. and Scott Samuel, A. *Research and Change in Urban Community Health*. Aldershot: Avebury, 57–66.

Springett, J., Costongs, C. and Dugdill, L. (1995) Towards a framework for evaluation in health promotion: the importance of process. *Journal of Contemporary Health* 2, 61–65.

Stevenson, H. and Burke, M. (1991) Bureaucratic logic in new social movement clothing: the limits of health promotion research. *Health Promotion International* 6(4), 281–289.

Strobl, J. and Bruce, N. (1997) *Report on the Evaluation of the Consultation Phase of Liverpool's Draft City Health Plan*. Liverpool: Urban Health Research and Resource Unit, University of Liverpool.

Taylor, J. (1997) *Monitoring the City Health Plan*. Liverpool: Liverpool Healthy City.

Tsouros, A. and Draper, R.A. (1993) The Healthy City Project: new developments and research needs. In Davies, J.K. and Kelly, M.P. (eds) *Healthy Cities: Research and Practice*. London: Routledge.

Weiss, C.H. (1988) Evaluation for decisions: is there anybody there? Does anybody care? *Education Practice* 9, 15–20.

WHO, Health and Welfare Canada and Canadian Public Health Association (1986) *Ottawa Charter for Health Promotion*. An International Conference on Health Promotion. Canada: Ottawa.

Willis, J. (1996) *Towards the Development of Proxy Indicators for the City Health Plan*. Liverpool: Liverpool City Council.

Winje, G. and Hewell, H. (1992) Influencing public health policy through action research. *Journal of Drug Issues* 22, 169–78.

Winter, R. (1990) *Action Research and the Nature of Social Inquiry*. Aldershot: Avebury.

Ziglio, E. (1991) Indicators of health promotion policy: directions for research. In Badura, B. and Kickbusch, I. (eds) *Health Promotion Research: Towards a New Social Epidemiology*. Copenhagen: WHO Regional Publications. European Series no. 37.

Chapter 10

Quality and effectiveness

International perspectives

Irving Rootman and Erio Ziglio

INTRODUCTION

Quality and effectiveness issues are critical in terms of the future of health promotion. Unless we can ensure the delivery of high quality and effective health promotion programmes and policies, health promotion is not likely to thrive in a climate that values efficiency and the 'bottom line', which increasingly appears to be the case in most countries. Thus, it is important that people working in health promotion at all levels pay attention to these matters.

This is one of the reasons that the European Office of the World Health Organization, with support from Canada (Health Canada), the United States (Centres for Disease Control and Prevention), and Europe (Health Education Authority England and the Finnish Ministry of Social Affairs and Health) established the WHO-EURO Working Group on Health Promotion Evaluation in 1995. Chaired by one of the authors of this chapter (Rootman), and consisting of members from Europe, Canada and the United States, its purpose was to increase the use, quality and appropriateness of evaluations of health promotion programmes and policies in developed countries.

To achieve this aim, it has reviewed current experience and commissioned background papers on evaluation issues in health promotion, sought and incorporated the views of policy-makers, practitioners and evaluators and produced reports, recommendations and guidelines aimed at key audiences. Although at the time of writing this chapter, the Working Group has not completed its work, sufficient progress has been made to enable us to identify key issues in the assessment of quality and effectiveness of health promotion interventions, and possible solutions. The latter will be elaborated in a book to be published by the European Office of the World Health Organization in 1999 (Rootman *et al.*, in preparation). This chapter will attempt to share what we have learned to date in relation to the topic of the present book – quality and effectiveness in health promotion.

In addition to drawing on the work of the Working Group, we will also draw on work on the Effectiveness of Health Promotion carried out by the

Centre for Health Promotion at the University of Toronto. In particular, we will use material presented at an international Symposium on the Effectiveness of Health Promotion in June 1996 (Dookhan-Khan, 1996) as well as activities following up on the symposium. This includes the work of three task groups – one on Evaluation, the second on Continuous Quality Improvement and the third on Consolidating Evidence on the Effectiveness of Health Promotion.

The chapter will first consider issues related to quality and then effectiveness in health promotion and will conclude with our reflections on where to go from here in relation to these matters, especially from an international point of view.

QUALITY ISSUES

There are many issues associated with an emphasis on 'quality' in health promotion. They include questions such as: Why consider quality in health promotion? What does quality mean? What are key areas for assessing quality? How should we set standards for measuring quality? What criteria should we use? How should we measure quality? What are the ethical considerations? These questions were addressed in a background paper prepared for the Working Group on Health Promotion Evaluation (Parish, 1996). Some of the same questions were addressed in a background paper on Continuous Quality Improvement for the Centre for Health Promotion Task Group in Health Promotion (Kahan 1998). She also identified a number of other questions which would need to be examined in order to assess the value of Continuous Quality Improvement (CQI) to health promotion. Some of the thinking in these two papers in relation to the questions follows in this section.

Why consider quality?

One of the key reasons why there has been a growing interest in quality in health promotion is related to the increasing concern about spiralling costs of health care. Since in most countries, health promotion is funded from the same budget as health services, 'there have been justifiable demands for health promotion to prove its worth' (Parish, 1996). In addition, the debate about health reform and the split between 'purchasers' and 'providers' in some countries, has added momentum to concern about quality in health promotion and to the demand to develop quality standards.

To this rationale for increasing interest in quality in health promotion, Kahan adds a perceived desire within the health promotion community to 'improve health promotion practice in order to increase the chances of achieving health promotion goals' (Kahan, 1998) as well as an expectation that governments will begin to require organizations that they fund to institute procedures for ensuring quality.

Thus, there are both external and internal reasons for people working in health promotion to at least think about quality in health promotion, even though it does make some people uncomfortable because it appears to reflect a paradigm and values which may be inconsistent with some of the core values of health promotion. In any case, both the WHO Working Group and the Centre for Health Promotion Task Group did proceed to look at quality in relation to health promotion.

What does quality mean?

In doing so, one of the first questions that they considered was what do we mean when we talk about quality? In discussing this issue, Kahan, citing Lethbridge *et al.* (1996), suggests that there seems to be some general agreement that 'quality embodies notions about efficiency, effectiveness and consumer satisfaction' (p. 2). She also suggests that a definition of quality take into account different viewpoints and be specific to health promotion and cites the three-tiered definition of quality put forward by Ovretveit (1996, p. 57) which differentiates between *consumer quality, professional quality* and *management quality*. She then discusses distinctions between Total Quality (TQ), Quality Assurance (QA) and Continuous Quality Improvement (CQI), focusing particularly on the difference between the latter two, suggesting that a key difference is the emphasis on a continuous process in CQI. On the other hand, Parish (1996) suggests that 'the whole notion of QA implies continuous evolution' and others (e.g. Simnett, 1995) have suggested that CQI and QA are complementary.

Whatever the case, it is clear that if we get into the quality business in health promotion we need to give as much, if not more emphasis, to process as to outcome. Furthermore, 'Quality thinking should pervade every aspect of health promotion, from planning to evaluation' (Parish, 1996). We would add that it needs to operate at all levels, from the international to the local.

What are key areas for assessing quality in health promotion?

In assessing quality in health promotion it is important to identify key areas on which to focus. Parish suggests that we look to the Ottawa Charter for Health Promotion (WHO, 1986) to identify the key processes which should underpin all health promotion work. In his view, these include: accountability; multi-sectoral action; community consultation; training and personal development; environmental action; organizational capacity; monitoring and evaluation; communications; equity; advocacy; enabling; and mediation. He further suggests that 'Quality will be achieved by setting standards in relation to these processes and by continuously measuring performance against them' (Parish, 1996).

Whether or not one agrees with this suggestion, that we use the Ottawa Charter as the framework for assessing quality and that the processes which he has identified are the key ones to measure, it is clear that we do need to specify what processes are particularly important from a health promotion point of view if we intend to try to measure quality. Certainly, his suggestion is a good starting point for doing so and is consistent with an international perspective on the matter.

How should we set standards for measuring quality?

There is some debate in the quality literature on the use of standards. According to Kahan, 'the argument against standards is that they are static, only looked at occasionally ... and ... they require only that a minimum be reached, so that groups have lowered aspirations' (Kahan, 1998, p. 7). On the other hand, others argue that there is a place for standards as long as they are continually upgraded. If such standards are used there are two dimensions to setting them: (1) specifying the level of performance in measurable terms; and (2) specifying the extent to which the standard will be met consistently (e.g. percentage of occasions). It is probably a good idea to start with a modest level of performance and raise the levels progressively. This would appear to us to be a prudent approach which will encourage health promotion practitioners to try harder and will indicate progress to those who are concerned about achieving the goals of the particular initiative.

In keeping with the emphasis on public participation in health promotion, we suggest that all the key stakeholders should be involved in the process of setting the standards to be achieved.

What criteria should we use?

We also suggest that the criteria should be determined in a participatory manner. Other stipulations are that criteria be precise, achievable, measurable, observable and reasonable (Evans *et al.*, 1994). Such criteria would be appropriate no matter what level we were working at.

How should we measure quality?

There are many different processes that might be undertaken to obtain the information required to measure quality, some of which have been outlined in this book. One approach is to create an audit tool or framework which usually consists of a number of questions to be asked in relation to each specified performance criterion. Others have outlined standard processes that might be applied. For example, McLaughlin and Kaluzny (1994) have suggested that CQI typically includes: a quality council; training programmes; mechanisms to select improvement opportunities; establishment of process improvement teams; staff support; and supportive personnel policies. Whatever the process, again we would recommend maximum possible participation by all concerned in the health promotion efforts being considered.

What are the ethical considerations?

There are a number of ethical issues and dilemmas that can occur in relation to efforts to assess quality in health promotion activities. One arises from the participatory approach that we have advocated. That is, it is possible that the various parties involved may hold diametrically opposed views which may constrain the extent of consultation or lead to pressure to use methods which may be viewed by some as unethical or ineffective. Another has to do with the lack of accepted procedures for reviewing ethical questions in relation to any particular quality assessment exercise. And a third has to do with the fact of multiple accountability which often exists and which may make it difficult to reach agreement on approaches to be used and ethical standards to be applied. All of these issues are a challenge for anyone involved in assessing quality and need to be addressed in a forthright, honest manner.

Other questions regarding CQI and health promotion

As mentioned earlier, Kahan (1998) also identified a number of other questions for judging the value of CQI to health promotion. They are:

- Is the philosophy of CQI compatible with health promotion principles, values and beliefs?
- Is CQI methodology and approach applicable to health promotion?
- If there are no irresolvable conflicts between CQI and health promotion, will implementing CQI processes improve health promotion practice and help achieve health promotion goals?
- If CQI is adaptable to health promotion, what would a CQI health promotion model look like?
- Are there options which would be better for health promotion than CQI (both in terms of improving practice and achieving goals)?
- Are there reasons not to implement CQI?
- What, if any are the consequences of implementing CQI?

She then makes an initial attempt to answer the questions.

With regard to the issue of compatibility, she makes the point that it depends on how the health promotion organizations define their principles, values and beliefs. That is, in some cases they may be compatible, and in others, not. In addition, compatibility may vary according to circumstances and some parts may be more compatible than others. On the other hand, there is some consensus developing on the principles, values and beliefs that characterize health promotion. For example, there is a growing agreement that health promotion should be defined using the definition of health promotion in the Ottawa Charter for Health Promotion as 'the process of enabling people to increase control over, and to improve, their health' (WHO, 1986). As suggested by the WHO Working Group, this implies that the primary criterion for determining whether or not a particular initiative should be considered to be of high quality ought to be the extent to which it brings about the *process of enabling or empowering* individuals or communities.

As for the applicability of the CQI methodology, she concludes that it is probably applicable, with some modifications and suggests some areas where CQI applied to health promotion may differ from CQI applied to other areas. For example, in the general literature, CQI tends to focus on the individual, whereas in health promotion, the focus is also on groups, communities or populations.

With regard to the third question, she suggests that CQI might increase empowerment of workers and community members, but thinks that more information is required before making a judgement. It may be useful in achieving some goals but not others.

In terms of a possible health promotion CQI model, she suggests that such a model might include the following steps:

- Define goals of the organization with reference to all constituents/constituencies
- Translate goals into desired outcomes
- Figure out measures/standards/benchmarks which would relate to the goals/outcomes
- Identify the processes currently being used to achieve the goals/outcomes
- Look at information from reports, studies etc. to see what different processes are being used by other organizations to achieve these, pinpointing the processes which come closest to achieving the desired goals/outcomes
- Figure out the possibilities – decide what to change and make sure to know how to tell what's an improvement and what isn't
- Implement – change the organization's processes to those more likely to achieve the desired goals/outcomes
- Document the implementation process
- Monitor results
- Make changes according to results
- Continue to review literature and what other organizations are doing; continue to review own results, and to make changes accordingly

Although these steps can be applied to most activities in both the public and private sectors, we suggest that in health promotion they need to be applied in a manner which is consistent with the key principles and values including especially empowerment and public participation. What is needed are pilot studies which would take these ideas and apply them in practice.

With regard to options that might be better than CQI, she notes that there is a range of 'best practices' approaches which might be considered. For example, one approach would be to rely strictly on evidence from the published literature related to randomized controlled trials. Another would be to include other published literature using other methods as well. Still another would be to include the personal experience of practitioners and policy-makers in a process of assessing 'best practices'. We recommend the latter, although we take the position that it is critical that assessment of 'best practices' be undertaken in as rigorous a fashion as possible given the source involved.

Kahan also identifies a number of reasons why some health promotion organizations might not want to implement CQI, including: time, money and commitment required; the effectiveness of CQI in health promotion has not been adequately documented; and some issues (e.g. indicators, appraisal methods) have not yet been worked out in a satisfactory manner.

On the other hand, however, she suggests that if health promotion does not adapt CQI or similar approaches to its own needs, a less compatible approach may be imposed by funders, and health promotion organizations may forfeit use of a method which might improve practice.

In sum, there are convincing arguments on both sides in terms of the value and compatibility of a CQI approach for health promotion – which suggests a certain level of caution before adopting such an approach fully. For this reason, the Centre for Health Promotion at the University of Toronto has decided not to proceed further with a CQI approach at the moment, but rather to explore the range of 'best practices' approaches. However, we will probably not have the luxury of avoiding the adoption of some kind of 'quality' approach for long.

In concluding this section of the chapter, it should be noted that the concepts and approaches to quality which we have been discussing here apply to research and evaluation as well as to programmes and policies. They also have relevance for people acting at all levels, from international to local. At the same time, it should be noted that the current policy and political environment in which the debate on quality in health promotion is taking place, may steer the search for quality in a direction and with methods that do not fit health promotion. In health promotion, quality can mean a totally different thing than it does in the private sector. Thus, we need to define quality in a way which is in line with the concepts and principles of health promotion. Furthermore, the assurance of quality in health promotion will have to be inventive and test a variety of new techniques and fora for dialogue and consensus building.

EFFECTIVENESS ISSUES

As is the case with quality, there are a number of key issues with regard to effectiveness in health promotion. They include: Why consider effectiveness in health promotion? What does effectiveness mean? What constitutes evidence of effectiveness in health promotion? What do we know about effectiveness in health promotion? What are key areas for further study? How should we proceed to study effectiveness? How do we consolidate evidence on the effectiveness of health promotion? How do we disseminate the evidence? What are the ethical considerations? Some answers to these questions have been suggested in the work of the Working Group on Health Promotion Evaluation and in the symposium and follow up activities of the Centre for Health Promotion and they will be presented in this section.

Why consider effectiveness in health promotion?

Although the WHO Working Group did not focus on effectiveness *per se*, it did discuss reasons why effort should be invested in evaluation in health promotion from the point of view of both the practitioner and the policy-maker. In terms of the former, Springett suggests that evaluation can help practitioners choose the appropriate programme, justify expenditures to funders, help them improve initiatives, contribute to knowledge development, develop networks and contacts, increase the legitimacy of health promotion activities, reflect on actions and improve standards (Springett, 1998). It also has an important role in empowering individuals and communities by informing people, providing a feedback mechanism and developing skills.

As for policy-makers, the WHO-EURO Working Group suggested that evaluation helps them: find out what works and how; make decisions about future health promotion policy strategies and programmes, but also about the role of health promotion in reaching broader policy goals; modify and improve current programs; justify policy choices; and increase the impact and effectiveness (including cost-effectiveness) of health promotion initiatives (WHO-EURO Working Group on Health Promotion Evaluation, 1998).

Many of these reasons also apply to the examination of effectiveness in health promotion. However, perhaps the overriding reason for being concerned about effectiveness in health promotion at this point in time is similar to the one noted in relation to quality. That is, concern with health care costs and opportunities related to health reform encourage us to put more effort and resources into looking at the extent to which health promotion efforts are able to achieve what they set out to achieve, or other worthy ends. Whether this is the main reason or not, there are certainly enough reasons for us to proceed along these lines.

What does effectiveness mean?

Springett, in her guidelines for practitioners, prepared for the WHO-EURO Working Group defined effectiveness as 'the extent to which stated goals and objectives are reached' (Springett, 1998). Similarly, the organizers of the international Symposium on the Effectiveness of Health Promotion defined it as: 'the extent to which an initiative was able to achieve its objectives or to produce short-term, intermediate or long-term positive outcomes' (Dookan-Khan, 1996, p. 1).

While we would not want to suggest that the latter is the definitive definition of effectiveness, it does have the merit of directing people to look at both process and outcomes in that the short-term outcomes would in fact probably be indicators of process. That is, the short-term outcomes correspond to 'instrumental processes', the intermediate-term to 'instrumental objectives' and the long-term to 'terminal goals'. In any case, the definition did help the authors identify what should be included in their assessments of the evidence on the effectiveness of health promotion. We will leave it to others, perhaps working together internationally, to produce the definitive definition of effectiveness, especially as it pertains to health promotion.

What constitutes evidence of the effectiveness of health promotion?

The question of what constitutes evidence of the effectiveness of health promotion initiatives was addressed by the WHO Working Group. Given the nature of health promotion initiatives which are often complex, changing and long-term, the Working Group suggested that it is difficult to argue that there is only one acceptable kind of evidence of effectiveness. Rather, the Group favours a pluralistic approach to evidence, one that finds value in both qualitative and quantitative data and in personal experience as well as research. Thus, one of the recommendations of the group to policy-makers is: 'Support the use of multiple methods to evaluate health promotion initiatives' (WHO-EURO Working Group on Health Promotion Evaluation, 1998). We are certain that most people working in health promotion would agree with this position, although there are no doubt policy-makers and researchers who would take issue with it and continue to put forward the randomized controlled trial as the 'gold standard'.

What do we know about effectiveness in health promotion?

The international Symposium on the Effectiveness of Health Promotion taught us that we, in fact, know a great deal about the effectiveness of health promotion initiatives. Moreover, other efforts to synthesize literature and experience on the effectiveness of health promotion (e.g. Hyndman, 1998a), including a number in this volume, have contributed to this knowledge. This is not the place to attempt to summarize this evidence, but simply to note that when it is put together, it adds up to an impressive endorsement of health promotion efforts. This is not to say that everything that we do in health promotion is effective – this is far from being true. However, it is to say that there is evidence of all kinds, ranging from RCTs to personal experience, which leads us to conclude that many of the activities that are carried out which fit with the WHO definition of health promotion, are effective and do have significant impact on the health and well-being of individuals and communities. Our task is to continue to document these successes (and failures as well) so that we can learn how to make what we do even more effective.

What are key areas for further study?

In doing so, it is clear that there are certain gaps in our knowledge which need to be filled on a priority basis. Since this chapter is intended to present international perspectives, we will limit ourselves to some of the things that we need to know about the effectiveness of health promotion at an international level. To this end, Makara (1996) suggests that the following are areas of priority action for increasing our knowledge regarding the evaluation of international partnerships:

- develop research activities on the quality of international co-operation;
- increase transparency of conflicting interest;
- increase focus on epistemology;
- analyse critically the use of auditing methods in international partnerships in health promotion;
- develop process evaluation techniques of partnerships, and tools indicating long-term sustainability of collaborative action; and
- launch international research on global co-operation in training and research for health promotion.

To these, we would add the following areas for priority attention:

- examine the policy environment for international health promotion initiatives;
- study the effectiveness of international projects and policies in health promotion; and
- analyse the main elements (such as quality and effectiveness) of capacity at local, national, international levels needed to sustain co-operation and partnership.

If implemented, all of these suggestions would take us a long way towards improving the effectiveness of international efforts in health promotion.

How should we proceed to study effectiveness?

As noted above, the Working Group suggested that a variety of methods and approaches are required in order to obtain evidence on the effectiveness of health promotion activities, many of which are considered in background papers which will be published by the European Office of WHO in 1999. More important than the individual methods however, is the adoption of a general approach consistent with the principles of health promotion. To this end, the Working Group has recommended that a 'participatory approach' be adopted in evaluating the effectiveness of health promotion efforts. This approach is spelled out in a paper released at the Fourth International Conference on Health Promotion (Rootman *et al.*, 1997) as well as in a set of guidelines prepared for practitioners by the WHO-EURO Working Group (Springett, 1998).

Briefly, it is suggested that evaluations in health promotion should cover the following steps:

- *Describe the proposed programme or initiative.* This includes clarifying the initiative's mandate, aims and objectives, linkage with other initiatives, procedures and structures. A programme logic model is often helpful in this process. It will also include getting people 'on board', establishing a group to oversee and undertake the evaluation, examining the health issues of concern, and collecting baseline information.
- *Identify the issues and questions of concern.* This would include deciding on the purpose(s) of the evaluation, clarifying the issues that are likely to be of concern to all of the stakeholders including the potential users of the evaluation, and specifying evaluation questions relative to the aims and objectives of the health promotion programme or other initiative. It is important that goals and objectives be clarified before deciding how to measure the extent to which they have been achieved. There is a danger that if measurement dictates the aims of an initiative, only quantifiable objectives will be pursued.
- *Design the process for obtaining the required information.* This includes deciding on the kind of evaluation to be carried out, the objects to be assessed, measurement methods, from whom the evaluation is undertaken, and when the data are to be collected. This step should also include choosing the best approach for the questions being asked as well as a plan for implementing the design. Achieving maximum participation in this process will ensure all experience is valued, and that information is collected from all credible sources.
- *Collect the data* by following the agreed-upon data collection methods and procedures.
- *Analyse and evaluate the data.* This includes interpreting the data, and comparing observed versus expected outcomes.
- *Make recommendations.* All the stakeholders should be involved in interpreting the results. This includes clarifying the short- and long-term implications of the findings, and identifying the costs and benefits of implementing and not implementing recommendations.

- *Disseminate findings.* This includes disseminating findings to funders, and to other stakeholders, in a meaningful and useful form.

These steps are iterative and, as Springett (1998) notes:

> At each stage there are a set of questions and key issues that need to be considered explicitly. These questions ensure that the aims of the project and the evaluation are clear, the objectives are set, the correct data are collected in the most appropriate way so as to measure the right outcomes in relation to the original objectives, all within the resources available.

We would add that all this has to be done in a context which is very dynamic and therefore challenging for the design of evaluations. Examples of the application of this approach are presented in Springett (1998).

The fact that the group is recommending a participatory approach does not eliminate the need for rigour in conducting studies on the effectiveness of health promotion. Whatever evaluation is carried out, should in fact be done so in as rigorous a fashion as possible consistent with the particular methodology being used. The group also suggests that, as far as possible, multiple methods be used.

How do we consolidate evidence on effectiveness of health promotion?

Given the many players who are and will continue to be involved in studying the effectiveness of health promotion efforts, it is important to develop means of assembling this diverse evidence in an organized and coherent fashion so that it can be shared with those who require it in a timely and appropriate manner. This is one of the issues that the Centre for Health Promotion Task Force on Consolidating Evidence in Health Promotion has been concerned about. Its main suggestion is that we attempt to develop a common framework for consolidating evidence on effectiveness and it has proceeded to do so. At the present time, this framework is in draft form (Hyndman, 1998b). The plan is to test it using a few areas of concern to health promotion (e.g. interventions to reduce poverty), to see whether or not it is viable and to make appropriate changes. Although this framework has been designed to be used in Canada, it may have applicability in other countries. In any case, it may be worthwhile to try to develop one at the international level.

How do we disseminate evidence on effectiveness?

Disseminating the evidence is another issue of concern to the Task Group on Consolidating the Evidence as well as to the WHO Working Group. While there is no easy answer to this issue, both groups feel that we need to invest more effort and resources in doing so. With the advent of computer technology, we are perhaps in a better position to be able to do so than we have ever been, although we need to pay attention to the fact that many of those who may need the information do not have ready use of such technology, at present, at least.

In any case, there is a need to explore innovative approaches to disseminating this knowledge, in addition to the more traditional approaches that have been used. In particular, there is a need to ensure that such knowledge reaches practitioners in an ongoing manner and appropriate form. Adopting a participatory approach may be helpful in this regard, but developing information vehicles directed specifically to this audience is also important.

What are the ethical considerations?

As was the case with 'quality', there are ethical considerations related to 'effectiveness'. Aside from the standard ethical issues that pertain to research in general, there are special ones associated with participatory approaches to research (Green *et al.*, 1995). One type of issue has to do with the potential harm that may come from community members being actively involved in research. Information that comes from such research might, for example, be used to discredit members of the community. Thus, it is important that safeguards are built into health promotion research to ensure that this doesn't happen. On the other hand, it is also important from an ethical point of view that procedures are built in to ensure open and honest communication among stakeholders when conducting participatory research. Unfortunately, appropriate structures which are able to review the special ethical issues associated with this kind of research have not generally been established.

Other issues

There are many other issues associated with the examination of the effectiveness of health promotion efforts including philosophical issues, conceptual issues, theoretical issues and political issues. Space, unfortunately, does not permit an exhaustive discussion here. For those who are interested, many of these issues are discussed in the paper released at the Fourth International Conference on Health Promotion (Rootman *et al.*, 1997) and in the forthcoming book (Rootman *et al.*, in preparation, Chapter 2) based on the work of the Working Group. Others are discussed in other chapters in this volume. We will, rather, conclude this chapter by reflecting on the issues that have been discussed and considering where to go from here, especially at the international level. Before doing so, however, we will briefly consider the relationship of 'quality' to 'effectiveness' as well as some conclusions that pertain to both.

QUALITY AND EFFECTIVENESS

Although we have dealt with 'quality' and 'effectiveness' separately in this chapter, it is quite clear that the two concepts are related to one another. For one, some of the issues are similar (e.g. ethical issues). For another, some of the recommended approaches (e.g. participatory) are the same. For a third, the underlying values that should govern our work in each of these areas is the same (e.g. empowerment). Many of the same courses of action recommended are the same (e.g. training). This should not be surprising given that some of the demand for both comes from the same sources and that they are complementary to each other; that is, it is impossible to assess or increase quality in health promotion without evidence regarding effectiveness. Similarly, it is impossible to study effectiveness without paying attention to quality. Thus, the two are inextricably intertwined and we need to constantly pay attention to both in our work in health promotion. To this end, the following are some observations and conclusions that apply to both quality and effectiveness in health promotion as drawn from a paper by one of the authors (Ziglio, 1997, pp. 29–32):

- We must be able to take up the opportunity to make evaluation of both effectiveness and quality of health promotion an integral part of health development. This means that we must understand the broader implications of our evaluative efforts. We must examine consequences that flow out beyond the immediate impact of an intervention on an individual or community. In other words, we have to look for the 'concentric ripples' emanating from our programmes or policies. It is these extant ripples of impact that will help us learn where we must make our next effort to strengthen the health quality process.
- There is a tendency in many countries to equate health promotion with behavioural and/or lifestyle changes. There is also confusion between behaviours and lifestyles. Furthermore, the ecological and environmental bases of health promotion are often disregarded (Chu, 1994). This tendency can steer the debate on quality only towards individual behavioural considerations. It would result in a rather limited and not too far-reaching and appropriate debate.
- For health promotion in the twenty-first century, our energy can be most productively applied to figuring out how this can be integrated effectively into mainstream social and economic development and have its influences visible in relevant programmes, regulations and wide-ranging public policies (Ziglio and Kretch, 1996). Searching for effectiveness and quality of health promotion could be assessed then against criteria that include matters of equity, empowerment, sustainability, accountability, acceptability, fiscal frugality, among others (WHO/EURO, 1995; 1996).
- We believe that contemporary health promotion has to focus primarily on population health rather than (only) individual health status. Health

promotion should increasingly work through large policy or programme initiatives with strong socio-ecological orientations. Thus, with health promotion being a new field of intervention, there is a pressing need for approaches to ensure quality that are uniquely appropriate to health promotion. In this endeavour, we must recognize that health promotion interventions are highly idiosyncratic and extremely sensitive to cultural and political contexts. We see this as an exciting challenge for health promotion. We must avoid pressures to passively adopt inappropriate approaches to building a 'quality based' health promotion.

CONCLUSION

In this chapter we have attempted to review key issues related to both quality and effectiveness in health promotion as reflected in the work of our WHO Working Group and the work of the Centre for Health Promotion at the University of Toronto. To summarize, in relation to quality, we have discussed the following issues: Why consider quality? What does quality mean? What are key areas for assessing quality in health promotion? How should we set standards for measuring quality? What criteria should we use? How should we measure quality? What are ethical considerations? There are other questions too, regarding Continuous Quality Improvement and health promotion. In relation to effectiveness, we have explored: Why consider effectiveness in health promotion? What does effectiveness mean? What constitutes evidence of the effectiveness of health promotion? What do we know about effectiveness in health promotion? What are key areas for further study? How should we proceed to study effectiveness? How should we consolidate evidence on the effectiveness of health promotion? How do we disseminate evidence on the effectiveness of health promotion? What are ethical considerations? We also considered the relationship between quality and effectiveness.

It is clear from what has been presented that there are a lot of issues that we need to be concerned about. At the same time, it is clear that they are not impossible issues to respond to in a positive and constructive manner. We have, in fact, made plausible suggestions for action in relation to each. We would like to conclude with some reflections on what might be done at the international level.

In terms of what might be done, the Working Group that we have drawn on is an excellent example of what can be accomplished with WHO's assistance. In fact, this initiative would probably not have taken place without WHO's involvement, in that WHO, through working with governments and national and local agencies in several countries, was able to assemble the resources required for the group. It is an example of international collaboration at its best, with all parties contributing according to their means under the umbrella of an international organization.

Having said that, there is more that WHO can do to further this enterprise. For example, once this Working Group has completed its work, WHO can solicit resources to develop models and processes for consolidating and disseminating evidence on both effectiveness and quality. It could also initiate an international effort to record intervention efforts including the contextual circumstances, strategies applied, logistical and technical aspects and observations of their impact. As has been suggested elsewhere, 'Without such a knowledge base, health promotion will lack the traction necessary to move forward towards a strategic theme that could guide its general advance and at the same time encourage national and regional variations' (Levin and Ziglio, 1996, pp. 33–40). As also noted by Levin and Ziglio (1996, pp. 33–40):

> The utility of the above-mentioned knowledge base should not be confused with the goal it serves: Namely, to lead toward the creation of a strategic approach to health promotion. Pursuing quality without such a strategic framework is something we do not recommend. The overall goal is, therefore, to document the synergistic contribution of its component parts to a holistic and equitable improvement in the health and well-being of the population. The focus should not be on documenting (evaluating) the impact and quality of isolated interventions as end points, but rather on the relationship of a given intervention to the other components of the health promotion strategy. Such an analysis may indeed provide a fresh approach to the very issue of quality.

In carrying out this work, WHO can use its extensive network of collaborating centres and others as resources and focal points. Even without additional resources, WHO can continue to offer leadership in this area by pressing the issues on the international stage through such mechanisms as the World Health Assembly.

However, we cannot rely on WHO alone to do all the work internationally. There are other international agencies and non-governmental organizations (e.g. the European Union, International Union for Health Promotion and Education, the World Bank, the Council of Europe, public health associations and similar organizations worldwide) that have a responsibility, to a different degree, in this area. Indeed, some of them are becoming increasingly interested in working in this area and have produced valuable material on effectiveness and quality assurance. In doing so, it is incumbent upon them to operate in a genuinely collaborative way with WHO and others who are interested in contributing. Similarly, governments that wish to help ought to do so collaboratively, as was done in the case of the Working Group.

At the same time, we need to recognize that contributing to the development of knowledge about effectiveness and quality in health promotion is not just the business of international organizations and governments. It involves us all, no matter where we are located. Each of us has a responsibility to do what we can to ensure that health promotion initiatives are of high quality and delivered in the most effective manner and that we learn from one another. There is no doubt that we are in a better position than ever to do so. All that is required is the will.

Note

The authors gratefully acknowledge the contributions of the members of the WHO-EURO Working Group on Health Promotion Evaluation as well as the Centre for Health Promotion Task Groups on the Effectiveness of Health Promotion. They also acknowledge the financial support of Health Canada, the Centres for Disease Control and Prevention, the Health Education Authority in England and Finnish Department of Social Affairs and Health and the Health Promotion Branch of the Ontario Ministry of Health.

References

Chu, C. (1994). Integrating health and environment: the key to an ecological public health. In C. Chu and R. Simpson (eds) *Ecological Public Health: From Vision to Practice*. Toronto: Centre for Health Promotion and ParticipACTION.

Dookhan-Khan, B. (1996). *The Proceedings of a Symposium on the Effectiveness of Health Promotion*. Toronto: Centre for Health Promotion, University of Toronto.

Evans, D., Head, M. and Speller, V. (1994). *Assuring Quality in Health Promotion*. London: Health Education Authority.

Green, L.W., George, M.A., Daniel, M., Frankish, C.J., Bowie, W.R. and O'Neill, M. (1995). *Study of Participatory Research in Health Promotion*. Ottawa: The Royal Society of Canada.

Hyndman, B. (1998a). *Health Promotion in Action: What Works? What Needs to be Changed?*. Toronto: Centre for Health Promotion, University of Toronto.

Hyndman, B. (1998b). *Framework for Consolidating Evidence on the Effectiveness of Health Promotion*. Toronto: Centre for Health Promotion, University of Toronto.

Kahan, B., (1998). *Continuous Quality Improvement*. Toronto: Centre for Health Promotion, University of Toronto.

Lethbridge, J. *et al.* (1996). *Quality and Health Promotion: Developing Concepts and Principles*. Proceedings of Second Meeting of European Committee for Health Promotion Development, Ormoz, Slovenia. Copenhagen: WHO Regional Office for Europe.

Levin, L. and Ziglio, E. (1996). Health promotion as an investment strategy: Considerations on theory and practice. *Health Promotion International*, 11(1), 33–40.

Makara, P. (1996). *International Partnerships for Health: Aspects of Evaluation*. National Institute for Health Promotion, Budapest.

McLaughlin, C.P. and Kaluzny, A.D. (1994). Defining total quality management. In McLaughlin, C.P., Kaluzny, A.D. (eds) *Continuous Quality Improvement in Health Care*. Gaithersburg, Maryland: Aspen Publishers, Inc.

Ovretveit, J. (1996). Quality in health promotion. *Health Promotion International*, 11(1), 55–62.

Parish, R. (1996). *Health Promotion: Towards a Quality Assurance Framework*. Background paper for WHO Workgroup. Copenhagen: WHO Regional Office for Europe.

Rootman, I., Goodstadt, M., Potvin, L., and Springett, J. (1997). *Toward a Framework for Health Promotion Evaluation*. Copenhagen: WHO Regional Office for Europe.

Rootman, I. *et al.* (eds). (in preparation) *Evaluation in Health Promotion: Principles and Perspectives*. Copenhagen: WHO Regional Office for Europe.

Simnet, I. (1995). Quality improvement and health development. In Simnet, I. *Managing Health Promotion: Developing Healthy Organizations and Communities*. Chichester: John Wiley and Sons.

Springett, J. (1998). *Guidance for Practitioners: The Evaluation of Health Promotion Initiatives*. Copenhagen: World Health Organization Regional Office for Europe..

WHO-EURO (1995). *Health in Social Development*. (WHO position paper, World Summit for Social Development, Copenhagen, March, 1995). Geneva: WHO.

WHO-EURO (1996). *Investment for Health in Slovenia*. Report of a team from WHO Regional Office for Europe and European Committee for Health Promotion Development. Copenhagen: WHO Regional Office for Europe, Health Promotion and Investment Office.

WHO-EURO Working Group on Health Promotion Evaluation (1998). *Health Promotion Evaluation: Recommendations to Policymakers*. Copenhagen: WHO Regional Office for Europe.

World Health Organization (WHO) (1986). *Ottawa Charter for Health Promotion*. Ottawa: Canadian Public Health Association.

Ziglio E. and Krech, R. (1996). Bruchenschlag zwischen politik und forschung in der gesudheitsforderung. In A Rutten and L. Rausch (eds) *Gesunde regionen in internationaler partnershaft: Konzepte und perspectiven*. Werbach-Gamberg, Germany: G. Conrad, Verlag fur Gesundheitsforderung.

Ziglio, E. (1997). How to move towards evidence-based health promotion interventions. *Promotion and Education* 1(2), 29–32.

Chapter 11

Beyond uncertainty

Leading health promotion into the twenty-first century

John Kenneth Davies and Gordon Macdonald

HEALTH PROMOTION: POST-OTTAWA OR THE THIRD MILLENNIUM?

This book has attempted to demonstrate that, despite growing evidence that health promotion is emerging as a discipline in its own right (Bunton and Macdonald 1992), it is still *striving towards certainties*, particularly in the area of effectiveness research and quality assurance programmes. Uncertainties are both a strength, allowing the flexibility to incorporate health promotion into various political ideologies, and a weakness, if it is perceived as a universal panacea. Before any decisions can be made about its effectiveness or quality, there is a need for international consensus on its meaning, relevant terminology and structures post-Ottawa Charter: 'Health promotion in its present form is riven with contradictions in theory and practice' (Kelly and Charlton 1995: 90).

This need for clarity applies not only to its detailed content, but also to the ideology, principles and values that underpin both health promotion research and practice. The underlying principles of Health for All, which lie at the heart of health promotion, regard access to good health as an equitable right for all, based on full participation, negotiation, community-defined need, empowerment and control by people over their own health and its determinants. There are numerous stakeholders involved in health promotion, each having their own expectations as to its scope and purpose. Each stakeholder, whether researcher, policy-maker, health professional, politician, funder or community activist, for example, has their own values and motivations regarding the goals and objectives of health promotion. It is crucially important therefore to clarify whose objectives are being pursued when carrying out assessment of quality and effectiveness. Attempts to evaluate or assess health promotion quality in its current state of development give rise to a wide range of uncertainties and challenges, as is evident in the content of contributions to this volume. Since the advent of the WHO/EURO Health Promotion Programme in the early 1980s, vehicles such as the Healthy Cities movement have been driven by practitioners, forever expanding upwards and outwards, with little time and resources being spent on theory and the development of strong research foundations

(Davies and Kelly 1993). Attempts were made early on to address key research questions and to reach some agreement internationally (WHO 1984; WHO 1985; WHO 1987), but these efforts were never followed up or pursued in any coordinated way until quite recently (see Rootman and Ziglio in this volume). Therefore the robustness of its research base has not allowed health promotion sufficient depth of analysis of programme processes and development to act as a sound basis for monitoring and evaluation. Is the failure of health promotion to move centre stage due to these uncertainties? Is it due to insufficient knowledge about what we are trying to do? Or having inadequate tools to measure activity? Or the failure to use both knowledge and tools appropriately?

PARADIGM WARS OR PARADIGM SHIFT?

Health promotion is defined as:

> a theory-based process of social change contributing to the goal of human development, building on many disciplines and applying inter-disciplinary knowledge in a professional, methodical and creative way.
>
> (Kickbusch 1997a: 267)

It is clear from this definition, by one of the founders of the health promotion movement, that health is perceived as a social phenomenon that is concerned with quality of life and social capital (Putnam 1993). Health promotion is a social movement, concerned with both individual and community-based reactions to social toxicity (the socially negative stressors and environments in which people live), particularly in terms of the processes and features of social organisation which facilitate collective action for mutual gain (Kickbusch 1997a). This analysis, presented at the Fourth International Conference on Health Promotion in Jakarta in 1997, provides a very different perspective of health promotion than that offered by traditional biomedical public health. The traditional view provides a rationale and logic which perceives health as an objective, measurable state and marginalises health promotion into an individual lifestyle education approach with undertones of moral regulation (Pederson and Lupton 1996).

Does this mean that we have rivalry between these two paradigms of health, or an incremental process of development from one paradigm to the other; a paradigm shift in our meaning and understanding about health? In this respect, new paradigms of health promotion theory and practice, defining health as a social phenomenon, have been perceived as having great resonance with postmodernism, providing a major epistemological challenge to our complex industrial societies and signalling the advent of the post-industrial era (Kelly *et al.* 1997).

In order to explore the eclectic theoretical basis for health promotion, it is useful to unpick and analyse these two paradigms as they form the basis of attempts to evaluate and assess quality. They reflect current dilemmas between the roles of public health medicine and health promotion, for example. The biomedical model perceives health in an individual, reductionist way as absence of illness, and regards health promotion or health education as a tool of preventive medicine, concentrating on behavioural risk factors. Effectiveness is based on predictability through repeatable, empirical results. Using the credibility of the medico-scientific paradigm it perceives effectiveness and quality only in positivist and empiricist terms; its gold standard being the randomised control trial. Its underlying ideology is expert driven, authoritarian and disempowering; seeking evidence through narrow clinically based methods and short-term quantitative outcome measures. Since the 1950s health education researchers, mainly in the United States, have developed numerous psychological models, based primarily on concepts of individual internal balance (subjective expected utility), in an attempt to understand and predict the way in which individuals make decisions about their health behaviour. No serious attention is given to the amelioration of socio-ecological or public policy factors. Using this approach, health education campaigns have sought to communicate messages from experts to target audiences, and have evaluated their actions through short-term measures of individual knowledge gain, attitude change and/or behavioural/lifestyle change (Bell *et al.* 1985).

Even more recent attempts have still tended to focus on similar, individual criteria (Driel and Keijsers 1997). Throughout this process, the target audience is perceived as passive receipients required to change in the recommended direction to achieve compliance. The methods used to monitor effectiveness and quality using this paradigm are based on quantitative, statistical techniques using experimental designs, borrowed from natural science. The limitations of this traditional approach, with its emphasis on victim-blaming, have been well documented. In research terms, attempts to isolate variables and assess their relationships has proven too simplistic and too narrow to provide the richness and diversity necessary to understand the complexity of health-related experience. Attempts to use these biomedical methods and measures to evaluate health promotion and assess its quality have proven to be uncomfortable and problematic. Yet, due to ever scarcer resources, we live in a world that is increasingly competitive. Does health promotion therefore have to tie in with the 'biologization of society' (Renaud 1993) and fit into the dominant paradigm to avoid being marginalised? '... potentially fruitful ventures like health promotion, if they have not been able to prove themselves in the terms defined by the biomedical world, are at risk of disappearing' (O'Neill *et al.* 1994: 385).

In the absence of more appropriate techniques, such dominant 'scientific' methods are being forced on health promotion in an effort to insist that it *proves* itself. This pressure from policy-makers, managers and clinicians, driven by economic rationalism and its associated value system, and lack of realistic understanding of intervention content, has not enabled health promotion to demonstrate its optimum potential.

A NEW PERSPECTIVE ON EFFECTIVENESS AND QUALITY?

As the methods, measures and indicators from biomedical, natural science perspectives are inappropriate, there is a need for a new toolbox which is more suitable to evaluate effectiveness and assess quality in health promotion. This was recognised in our first chapter of this book, but we would like to elaborate here. What are the contents of such a new toolbox?

Effectiveness

In research terms, the emphasis on psychological approaches, referred to above, has resulted in a dearth of work on the socio-ecological context or 'settings' in which people live, particularly in relation to socio-cultural factors and processes of healthy public policy development.

Focus on process measures

The dynamic nature of health promotion involves a complex interplay of processes in complex social systems (Noack 1997), which means that it is time and location specific and inappropriate to be based on a narrow predictive model, such as that offered by the biomedical paradigm. The immediate outcomes of health promotion should be to establish favourable conditions to promote health, allow participation and empower people. Therefore, process is more important than outcome. Such processes need to be identified, monitored and measured. There is a need for collective health status measures and the ability to measure community empowerment in process terms, not just by aggregating individual responses. In other words, the value-added benefits of a sense of coherence among social groups and their collective action for mutual health gain through the growth of supportive social environments (Kickbusch 1997b). We need to understand more clearly the complex social processes and relationships that underlie health (social capital) and see them as valuable outcomes in their own right (see Speller *et al.* and also Haglund *et al.* in this volume). Setting the processes of programme planning and implementation within their socio-ecological context, would aid understanding to evaluate effectiveness and *improve* quality. Continous quality improvement is therefore more relevant to post-Ottawa Charter health promotion.

Research methodology

We need to utilise more appropriate research approaches, using interpretative and process-based methods, which aid knowledge development, and qualitative constructivist methods, which provide individually meaningful views of reality. Along with participatory research, such approaches fit most appropriately with the principles underpinning health promotion.

Role of the researcher

Health promotion is a value driven activity. The values held by health promotion researchers and evaluators, along with their disciplinary training, will influence the methods and instruments they choose to use. Are health promotion researchers therefore activists, seeking to bring about improvements in health; working as facilitators and interpreters, perhaps using participatory methods to empower people?

Appropriate tools and instruments

There are still uncertainties regarding the most appropriate techniques and measures. It is proposed that the action areas of the Ottawa Charter serve as foci for new indicators of effectiveness and quality related to its underlying Health for All values. There is a need to create new criteria and indicators more related to structural and environmental change, particularly in relation to community organisation and the settings in which people live. Our understanding of these processes and their effects is in its infancy with regard to health promotion.

Some suggested new measures and approaches which build on ideas raised in our earlier chapter, and indeed by other contributors to this volume, are:

- *Intermediate indicators*: proxy input measures set within the assessment of policies (number of health promotion sessions, training of personnel) and intermediate indicators (related to process such as changes in knowledge and attitudes)
- *Participative needs assessment*: within the community the use of focus groups and rapid appraisal techniques for community profiling
- *Storytelling*: not just to describe how and when events happened, but why; the use of reflection and experiential learning approaches

Quality as a way of improving practice

Quality as a form of continous improvement has gained popularity in recent years and as a participative process fits with the ideology of health promotion. It should be a fundamental part of the assessment of the planning and implementation process and utilised as a way of assessing practice as a whole. Quality needs to be built into these preparatory and operational stages as a form of pre-testing (for example, in this volume, the use of the SESAME measurement instrument in Haglund *et al.*, and the use of action research methods as a core part of policy development in Springett).

Quality as a way of testing standards

The instruments offered by Haglund *et al.* and Keijsers and Saan, in this volume, are useful starting points for the development of QA instruments and help form a core part of policy development, using similar techniques to action research methods (see Springett).

Participation and empowerment

There is a core weakness in most of the current attempts at quality development work in that they are still normatively or professionally driven. This is highlighted and readily acknowledged in this volume, for example, by Speller *et al.* The participative and empowering ideology of health promotion provides a continual tension between the community and professionals, institutions and their power structures. Whose needs are being met? Priority is given to the establishment of professional standards, mainly by national health promotion agencies or government bodies. It is questionable whether these moves will enhance the empowering nature of health promotion, or simply reinforce the status quo with power and control in the hands of professionals. Effectiveness and quality assurance cannot be separated from the ideological and political basis of health promotion. Involvement by members of the community and wider community perspectives are urgently needed. Innovative attempts, with relevant evaluation methods and indicators, are being tested through new community-based approaches (see, for example, the work of Baum in this volume). What is now needed is criteria of enablement which focus on the means for participation in line with the thinking behind the Ottawa Charter.

Recommendations

The reality is that we will probably have to exist in no man's land between these two paradigms for well into the twenty-first century – a situation reflected in the contributions to this volume. Yet we need agreement on how to proceed to maintain clear water and a fertile environment for the contents of the new toolbox to be developed. This should allow health promotion to progress, without being hijacked by the battalions of biomedicine or playing a subordinate role to public health medicine.

Below are seven ideas which we feel will help to move health promotion to the heart of health development worldwide:

1   *Development of a pluralistic framework or taxonomy for health promotion*: this will help in assessing effectiveness and quality, with common underlying principles, a sound theoretical base, a common terminology (the revised version of the WHO health promotion glossary acts as a sound

basis for work on developing such common terminology (WHO 1998a), and a set of criteria and code of practice for setting appropriate standards. This should include short-term outcomes, as indicators of process, and guidance on the effective use of both qualitative and quantitative methodologies.

The integrative and functional role played by the health promotion researcher should be acknowledged – validity, objectivity and reliability being replaced by credibility, transferability and dependability. Phenomena are explored in their natural setting. An inductive approach is taken to data analysis, which focuses on process and stresses the meaning people give to their experiences (Bogdan and Biklen 1982). Such approaches to research provide a greater understanding of the context in which health promotion occurs, by exploring meanings and processes in depth.

2   *More experience in use and demonstration of appropriate intervention strategies and complementary evaluation and quality assurance processes*: health promotion activities are unique in terms of intervention, time, place and people. They are dynamic and process related and therefore unpredictable. We need to continuously review them, examining quality and effectiveness at each stage of preparation, planning and implementation.

3   *Better communication and dissemination*: more extensive networking and sharing of experiences of good practice are needed. Currently, there is little discussion, publication and dissemination of these issues. There is a need for better communication, not only between researchers and practitioners, but with policy-makers, and not least, between health promoters themselves. This relates to a requirement for sharing experiences from local projects and disseminating good practice. Dedicated clearing houses, utilising the latest communication technology, need to be established internationally to facilitate such dissemination. The Internet is sadly underdeveloped in this area; although initiatives such as the Health Promotion and Disease Prevention Research Network (from Karolinska Institute, Sweden) and the *Internet Journal of Health Promotion* (Griffith University, Australia) are to be commended for their work. The creation of quality review networks would be a positive move. One of the key recommendations of the Turin Conference supported the establishment of a European Regional Quality Review Network. This would help with the sharing of experiences and standardisation of databases.

4   *Better coordination*: we need to consolidate evidence on effectiveness, but who takes the lead on this? We have seen what cooperation can achieve between a UN agency working with expert and financial support from interested national agencies – the WHO work group (Rootman and Ziglio in this volume). But better cooperation is required urgently, especially between international agencies, to plan cooperatively in the key areas of research and training in health promotion, especially in the sharing of expertise and resources.

5   *Better research and development:* more experience is required in the use and demonstration of appropriate intervention strategies and the complementary evaluation and quality assurance processes. Specific research is needed in order to achieve excellence in terms of boosting knowledge with regard to:

    • programme/intervention settings
    • changing socio-cultural and environmental factors
    • processes of healthy public policy
    • exploration of dedicated underlying theory eg salutogenesis, and relating theory to practice
    • social processes and ways collectives and organisations relate to social toxicity
    • community empowerment and processes of collective social support

6   *Better training:* in order to produce standards of quality in terms of applying theory into practice. This could be developed, for example, from training initiatives in Europe, initiated under the health promotion programme of the European Commission; in the Americas by the Pan-American Health Organisation (PAHO) and from inter-regional discussions during conferences such as the World Conference of the International Union for Health Promotion and Education. Such initiatives encourage better communication between universities on standards in education and training and endorse the need to produce skilled, competent practitioners.

7   *Better attempts at community links:* a lack of 'consumer', or perhaps more appropriately 'community', involvement in health promotion may lead to the danger of paternalism by professionals. Is the concept of quality supported by values consistent with those of the Ottawa Charter for health promotion? The literature may divide quality into professional, management and consumer segments or perspectives, but does the 'consumer' actually have a view or say in programme planning or delivery? Who actually sets standards of quality? Is it only related to efficiency criteria or to cost and benefit? When does the individual 'consumer' or community set standards? Does the current professionally dominated system seek to empower individuals or communities, or simply develop a new 'mask' of respectability by evolving new measures of assurance that leave the user or consumer even more confused and powerless. Our challenge is to ensure this does not happen through the techniques of real participation in the planning, implementation and evaluation of programme effectiveness and quality. Only then can we be sure that the evidence we collect is based on people certainty.

By collaborative effort internationally, focused on these seven areas, the powerful ideas and actions offered by the post-Ottawa health promotion movement can be strengthened and given credibility in terms of effectiveness and quality as we approach the third millennium. Thereby health promotion can be accepted, to quote the 1998 Health Promotion Resolution of the Executive Board of WHO, as 'a "key investment" and an essential element of health development' in the twenty-first century, making significant changes to our understanding of health and offering the potential to tackle the growing inequalities in health (WHO 1998b).

References

Bell, J. Billington, D.R., Macdonald, M., Drummond, N. and Thompson, G. (eds) (1985) *Annotated Bibliography of Health Education Research Completed in Britain from 1979–1983*. Edinburgh. Scottish Health Education Group.

Bogdan, R.C. and Biklen, S.K. (1982) *Qualitative Research for Education: an Introduction to Theory and Methods*. Boston. Allyn and Bacon.

Bunton, R. and Macdonald, G. (eds) (1992) *Health Promotion: Disciplines and Diversity*. London. Routledge.

Davies, J.K. and Kelly, M.P. (eds) (1993) *Healthy Cities: Research and Practice*. London. Routledge.

Driel, W.G. van and Keijsers, J.F.E.M. (1997) An instrument for reviewing the effectiveness of Health Education and Health Promotion. *Patient Education and Counselling* 30, 7–17.

Kelly, M. and Charlton, B. (1995) The modern and the postmodern in health promotion. In Bunton, R., Nettleton, S. and Burrows, R. *The Sociology of Health Promotion: Critical Analyses of Consumption, Lifestyle and Risk*. London. Routledge: 78–90.

Kelly, M., Davies, J.K. and Charlton, B. (1997) Healthy cities: a modern problem or a postmodern solution? In Sidell, M., Jones, L., Katz, J. and Peberdy, A. (eds) *Debates and Dilemmas in Promoting Health*. Basingstoke. Macmillan/The Open University: 353–362.

Kickbusch, I. (1997a) Think health: what makes the difference? *Health Promotion International* 12(4): 265–272.

Kickbusch, I. (1997b) Health promoting environments: the next steps. *Australian and New Zealand Journal of Public Health* 21(4): 431–434.

Noack, H. (1997) Research for health promotion: a challenge for the 21st century. Paper prepared for the 4th International Conference on Health Promotion, Jakarta, Geneva, World Health Organization.

O'Neill, M., Rootman, I. and Pederson, A. (1994) Beyond Lalonde: two decades of Canadian health promotion. In Pederson, A., O'Neill, M. and Rootman, I. (eds) *Health Promotion in Canada: Provincial, National and International Perspectives*. Toronto. W. B. Saunders: 374–386.

Pedersen, A. and Lupton, D. (1996) *The New Public Health: Health and Self in the Age of Risk*. London. Sage.

Putnam, R. D. (1993) The prosperous community: social capital and public life. *The American Prospect*, spring: 35–42.

Renaud, M (1993) Social science and medicine: Hygeia versus Panakeia. *Health and Canadian Society* 1: 229–247.

WHO (1984) *World Health Organization/Scottish Health Education Group Workshop on Research in Health Promotion*. Edinburgh WHO/EURO.

WHO (1985) *World Health Organization Working Group on Research in Health Promotion*. Copenhagen. WHO/EURO.

WHO (1987) *World Health Organization/Scottish Health Education Group/Research Unit on Health and Behavioural Change*. University of Edinburgh Symposium on the New Public Health: Implications for Research. Edinburgh. WHO/EURO.

WHO (1998a) *Health Promotion Glossary*. Geneva. World Health Organization.

WHO (1998b) *Health Promotion Resolution*. The Executive Board of the World Health Organization, 101st Session, 24 January 1998. Geneva, World Health Organization.

Author index

Subject index